Hello, Methuselah!

LIVING TO
100
AND BEYOND

George Webster

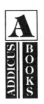

Addicus Books, Inc.
Omaha, Nebraska

An Addicus Nonfiction Book

ISBN# 1-886039-25-9

Cover design by George Foster

Illustrations by John Ritland

Typography by Linda Dageforde

Library of Congress Cataloging-in-Publication Data

Webster, George, 1924-
  Hello, Methuselah! : living to 100 and beyond / by George Webster.
    p.   cm.
  Includes bibliographical reference and index.
  ISBN 1-886039-25-9 (alk. paper)
  1. Longevity. I. Title.
QP85.W385 1997
612.6'8—DC21   96-39083
                                                              CIP

Addicus Books, Inc.
P.O. Box 45327
Omaha, Nebraska 68145
e-mail: AddicusBks@aol.com
Web site: http://members.aol.com/addicusbks

Printed in the United States of America

10 9 8 7 6 5 4 3 2 1

To Sandy

Contents

Acknowledgments

I am grateful to many people who contributed to the development of ideas in this book. I especially thank Kimberley Bourne, M.D., for continually taking time for her busy schedule to advise me about diseases and their treatment. I also profited from discussions with more researchers than I can possibly list, but particularly from those with Charles Polson, Ph.D., Florida Institute of Technology; Arlan Richardson; Ph.D., Audie Murphy VA Hospital; Raj Sohal, Ph.D., Southern Methodist University; Richard Sprott, Ph.D., National Institute on Aging; Bernard Strehler, Ph.D., University of Southern California; Roy Walford, M.D., University of California at Los Angeles; and Jeffrey Webster, Ph.D., National Institute for Environmental Health Sciences.

My work would not have been possible without support from the American Federation for Aging Research, the Gannett Foundation, Saul Kent and the Life Extension Foundation, the Don and Charity Yarborough Foundation, the National Institutes of Health, and the National Science Foundation.

I also express my heartfelt thanks to Susan Adams and Rod Colvin for editorial guidance and encouragement in the preparation of this book.

Introduction

*Anything that is theoretically possible will be achieved
in practice, no matter what the technical difficulties,
if it is desired greatly enough.*
—Arthur C. Clarke, *Profiles of the Future*

A lmost everyone wants to live longer. I learned this as
soon as I began to do research on what causes aging.
My university regularly reported to the media on research by
our professors. Work by my colleagues on the sex life of
squiggly things or the beauty of pond scum only got yawns
from reporters. But if we discovered anything about aging, all
hell broke loose. We got television cameras. We got the
press. We got clogged phone lines. We got an avalanche of
letters and an office full of people wanting to live forever. I
didn't have to be very bright to see that living longer is a hot
topic.

So, I did an informal experiment. When I gave public
lectures on aging, I asked this question.

"If you could be healthy and active, would you like to
live for 300 years?"

More than 95 percent said, "Yes!" Most not only wanted
to live for 300 years, but many also wanted to live forever.
When you think about it, that isn't surprising. Our strongest
instinct is to stay alive. Writings throughout history, from
Genesis to James Hilton's classic novel, *Lost Horizon*, express the human dream of long life, even immortality.

"Whoa!" you say. "Live for 300 years? Impossible!"

That same feeling pervaded my audiences. They wanted to live for 300 years but were certain it is impossible. To a scientist, there is nothing impossible about it. Something is impossible only if it violates a physical law. This is a basic tenet of science. Living for 300 years doesn't violate a physical law, so it has always been possible. It is a human failing to think that something we haven't yet done is impossible. Instead of following facts to a logical conclusion, we too often follow our intuition, which tells us that the earth is flat and that a heavy object like an airplane can't possibly fly.

When I was at CalTech in the 1950s, I heard a lecture by Dr. Wernher von Braun, the rocket pioneer. He described how humans could fly through space to land on the moon and the planets.

"Impossible!" I thought. "This is Buck Rogers stuff."

I couldn't believe he was serious. At the time, the United States had launched few rockets. I'd watched on television as most of them exploded spectacularly.

Fifteen years later, on a hot morning in July, I stood in bright sunshine on the roof of my laboratory building at Cape Canaveral, Florida. Several miles behind me was a crowd as vast as all the Super Bowls combined. A million persons were on hand, and millions more watched on television. In front of me, a Saturn rocket rose with a thunder that shook the ground. It lifted an Apollo spacecraft on its way to land on the moon. From "impossible" to success took 15 years.

Why the big change in so few years? Space flight violated no physical law, so it was possible. Success came from dividing the problem of going to the moon into smaller problems, breaking those into still smaller problems, and then solving each.

Today, it's just as difficult for many to accept the idea of a 300-year life as it was for people in the 1950s to accept travel to the moon. For example, just a few years ago, a scientist told the media that we can't expect to live past 85. Today, people living past 85 are our fastest-growing age group. More recently, an elderly gerontologist wrote that 115 is the absolute limit for human life. The many persons who have now lived beyond 115 must find his statement puzzling. There is no evidence of a limit to how long we can live.

More important, biomedical science is moving us toward a 300-year life span at an ever faster pace. We are further along than you may think. Today, for the first time in history, health-conscious adults can expect to live 100 years. The U.S. Census Bureau reports an astonishing increase in the number of people living past 100.

You may have read that we can only expect to live an average of 76 years. That is misleading. Seventy-six is what you can expect if you are a newborn baby. A 35 year-old can expect to live to 78, and a 65 year-old to 82. Why? Because they have already overcome many hazards that a newborn must face. Even 78 and 82 are deceptive because they are averages for the entire United States, including an estimated 40 million smokers, 10 million drug users, a million AIDS victims, a million illegal aliens, and millions of couch potatoes, all averaging lives shorter than 76. If you are a health-conscious person—a non-smoker who exercises, eats a healthful diet, and uses all medical means to keep fit—you can expect to live past 100.

Today's 100 years is a milestone for the human dream of long life. Future generations will look back on it as a harbinger of things to come, because 100 is only the beginning. If research advances at its present rate (and all evidence suggests it will), we will be able in coming decades to extend human life past 100 to 150, 300, and beyond. This is of enormous importance because it will affect us more profoundly than anything else in history. Scholars predict vast effects on our economy, society, and personal life. It will transform our populace, business, employment, retirement, insurance, family, education, and nearly everything else. Above all, it will affect you personally. How do you feel about 150 years, 300 years, or an unlimited span of healthy, active life?

We always seem unprepared for science's latest leap forward. Before an advance, people scoff at the possibility, only to be stunned when it occurs. Yet, to a scientist, there are clear signs of what is coming. For example, when polio held the nation in its grip, the media was gloomy about an end to the death and the paralysis of its pitiful victims, especially children. At the time, my lab at CalTech was across the hall from that of Renato Dulbecco, later a Nobel laureate, who was doing work on the polio virus. Just from the chatter drifting across the hallway it was clear that a vaccine was coming. I'm sure virologists knew it, but when it came, it stunned the world. Scientists get wind of coming advances in many ways. They put together the findings in many reports, often obscure, in scientific journals. They hear of them at scientific meetings. They pick up gossip. They browse the Internet, which buzzes with exciting new information.

This is my reason for writing this book. As a molecular biologist, I see evidence everywhere of a rapid movement to extend healthy human life to astonishing lengths. It's high time we talk of it.

I wrote this book for non-scientists. Although everything in it is based on hard science, it is not a scientific treatise. A great problem in our society is the failure of scientists to communicate clearly with people outside the world of science. This has hurt support for science and, as Carl Sagan said in *The Demon-Haunted World*, has let pseudoscience grow to an alarming degree. This book is for those of you who want to know how we are extending life but are put off by incomprehensible scientific talk.

This book is two things. First, it's a no-nonsense guide

to living 100 healthy, active years *today*. Second, it's a view ahead along the rising trends of discoveries toward the conquest of diseases and aging. They are already coming into view. When you reach them, you will be as close to immortality as it is possible to get. Ready? Let's go!

1

Thinking the Unthinkable

Let's give everyone a 300-year life.
How valuable life would be if it lasted for 300 years!
— Karel Capek, *The Makropoulos Secret*

L et's begin by considering how we can extend life. From the standpoint of science, it is simple. We extend life by identifying the things that kill us and by getting rid of them. Diseases kill us. Accidents kill us. Aging kills us. Whether it's 100 years today or 300 years tomorrow, we live longer every time we:

- Prevent diseases and accidents,
- Cure the diseases we don't prevent, and
- Control aging.

At first glance, it seems unbelievable that we could overcome these barriers to longer life. But if we analyze them, they aren't nearly as formidable as they appear. Each is big, but we don't try to solve them all at once. We do what the engineers did to go to the moon. We divide the big problems into smaller problems, divide those into still smaller ones, and then solve each.

When people think of living longer, they usually think of halting aging, as happened when the people in James

Hilton's *Lost Horizon* entered the valley of Shangri-la. But if researchers tomorrow discovered a drug to stop aging, unconquered disease would go right on killing us. The prevention and cure of diseases is just as important as the control of aging. The number of diseases is limited. Again, it may seem unbelievable, but at the rate medicine is advancing we should be able to prevent or cure essentially all of them in the twenty-first century. We can't keep moving forward rapidly without eventually reaching our goal. Just one hundred diseases cause 99.9 percent of all deaths. Thus, each time we learn how to prevent or cure another disease, we will extend life. Research today is working to conquer all one hundred, plus many more.

But if we live longer by overcoming diseases, aging will still kill us. To live 300 years, we must not only overcome diseases but also control aging. We are far along in doing just that in the laboratory.

The History Of Major Diseases

In Greek and Roman times, life expectancy was 20-25 years. It was little better than the 15 years estimated for early man. If we date human civilization from about 3000 B.C., life expectancy has been 20-25 years for most of our time on earth. Our ancestors had pitiably short lives.

Life expectancy was 20-25 years because of the towering barriers to longer life. The first was smallpox, the primary cause of death for centuries, going back to our earliest history. One was almost certain to get it, often at birth, and it killed half of those infected. Even in the 1700s, it killed 60 million Europeans, plus millions in Asia, Africa, and the Americas. Survivors were usually disfigured and often blinded by the disease. If one eluded smallpox, other barriers blocked the way to longer life. Bubonic plague killed 90-100 percent of those infected. When it spread across Europe in 1347, 24 million people died. It hit again in 1361 and 1369, killing another 20 million. By 1400, a third of Europe's population had died from the plague. In the same period, it nearly wiped out the entire population of China. If one got past smallpox and the plague, longer life was often halted by tuberculosis (consumption), typhoid, cholera, diphtheria, or a dozen other diseases that constantly infected the population and killed millions.

Imagine a long, dark road leading to the dawn of immortality. If you had lived before 1700, you likely could have moved only 20-25 years along the road because your way was blocked by the massive barrier of smallpox. If you had surmounted this barrier, you probably would have lived longer. Your way would have been blocked by yet another barrier, perhaps bubonic plague. Each time you overcame a barrier, you lived longer, only to face yet another disease. We still travel this road today, but the end is just becoming visible—far ahead, but in sight.

The salvation for mankind was the rise of science. Scientists demand absolute proof of any claim before they accept it as a fact, and so should you. Today, we still have people, some charlatans and some well-meaning, who tout all kinds of unproven cures for diseases or aging. If we believe them, without proof, we are no further advanced mentally than primitive man.

Before 1700, physicians were helpless against diseases because scientific medicine did not exist. The accepted practices were to give patients herbal brews, hang amulets around their necks, induce diarrhea with purges, and drain their blood. Barbers performed surgery with no knowledge of sterility, so patients died in droves from infected wounds. The 1700s saw the start of primitive medicine and hygiene based on science. The life expectancy was raised to 27 by 1800. The foremost barrier to longer life fell in 1798, when Dr. Edward Jenner discovered how to prevent smallpox. The control of rats broke the barrier of the bubonic plague. The finding that bacteria cause a multitude of diseases led in the late 1800s, to a search for preventive methods. These, together with drugs, hygiene, sterile surgery, and progress in medicine, almost doubled life expectancy from 27 in 1800 to 47 in 1900.

Still, in the United States in 1900, one in five children died before age 6. Almost 40 percent of people died before age 30. The leading barriers to longer life then were:

- Pneumonia/Influenza
- Tuberculosis
- Typhoid/Cholera
- Cardiovascular Disease
- Accidents

- Stroke
- Measles
- Scarlet Fever
- Cancer
- Diphtheria

Six of these barriers are infectious diseases. They were a top priority for research in the early 1900s. Figure 1-1 shows what has happened to each.

Pneumonia has fallen to sulfa drugs, antibiotics, and immunization. It has slipped from being the leading cause of death in 1900 to sixth place in 1990. It would be lower if everyone were immunized. Tuberculosis has yielded to quarantines, drugs and antibiotics. It nearly vanished, but it has returned among illegal aliens, drug addicts, and AIDS victims. Typhoid and cholera have succumbed to immunization and public health measures for pure water, milk, and food. Diphtheria has been wiped out by immunization. Antibiotics have eliminated scarlet fever. Measles has declined steadily due to immunization.

As a result, life expectancy in the United States has risen from 47 in 1900 to 76 in 1996. It is 77 in Australia, France, Norway, and Spain; 78 in Canada, the Netherlands, Sweden, and Switzerland; and 79 in Japan. Beginning with smallpox, the removal of barriers to longer life has quadrupled life expectancy.

Notice the trend in Figure 1-2, which shows life expectancy in developed nations. The period just before 1700 marks the end of thousands of years of life expectancy near age 20. In the past 300 years, the trend has curved sharply

Figure 1-1. Conquest of Infectious Diseases

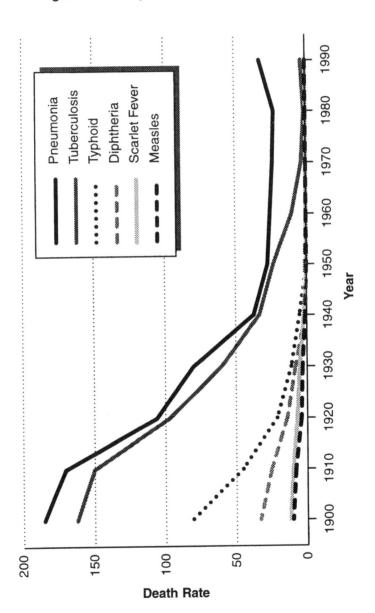

upward. It projects a rise in life expectancy of the populations of developed nations to age 150 by the year 2100. The
life expectancy of health-conscious people will be 150 long
before the year 2100, however. Their longevity will quickly
curve upward to 110, 120, or 130. As we control aging, it
will climb to astounding levels. Many will still be living in
2100.

Figure 1-2. Life Expectancy (1200-1990)

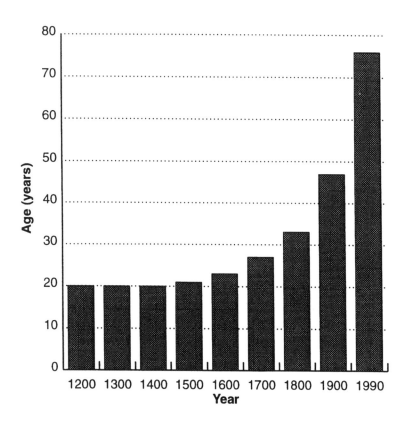

Barriers Today

The past teaches us that we boost life expectancy by conquering the immediate barriers to longer life. Many improvements in medicine and public health have extended life, but longer life has come mainly through the conquest of infectious diseases. As we move into the twenty-first century, people will live longer than ever before. Yet we will face a new set of barriers, not from infectious diseases but instead from poor health habits, the environment, and genes.

Figure 1-3 shows cardiovascular disease and cancer are the biggest barriers to longer life today. Behind them, stroke, chronic lung disease, and accidents are major obstacles. Pneumonia and diabetes, although deadly, are lower

Figure 1-3. Leading Causes of Death

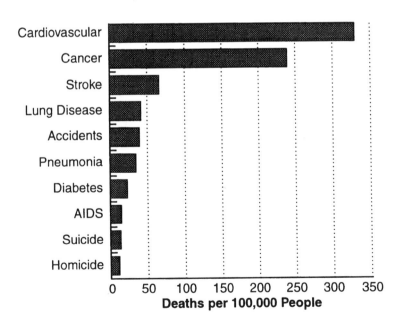

Deaths per 100,000 People

hurdles because they are both preventable or treatable. AIDS, suicide, and liver disease are still lower barriers, although they kill thousands each year. The diseases seem daunting, but they are no more so to scientists now than pneumonia, tuberculosis, and typhoid were to scientists in 1900. We are advancing rapidly against all these barriers, extending life further.

Today's Rising Longevity

Our escalating ability to overcome today's barriers to longer life is not abstract. It strikes us personally. It's not your imagination that there seem to be more older people around or that they seem more active. In 1990 the U.S. Census Bureau found that the number of people over 65 had more than doubled since 1950 and had jumped from 25 million to 31 million people in the single decade of the 1980s. Even more striking is the rise in the number of people living past 85 and especially beyond 100. The number of persons over 85 is growing six times faster than any other age group. Figure 1-4 shows what is happening in the United States. In the early 1900s, few persons lived beyond 85. Then, in the 1960s and 1970s, the number of people living past 85 rose 30 percent each decade. That, however, was nothing compared with the 1980s. In that single decade, the number of people over 85 almost doubled. The U.S. Census Bureau expects those living past 85 to nearly double again by 2000. Note how the bars in Figure 1-4 curve upward. This rising curve forecasts a huge rise in the number of people living beyond 85 in the coming years.

Another sign of rising longevity is the many persons living past 90. By 1991, more than a million people in the United States were 90 years or older, with the number growing 42 percent since 1981. If the climb continues (and all evidence suggests it will), 90-year-olds in 2000 will be as numerous as 80-year-olds were in 1980.

Figure 1-4. People Living Beyond 85 and 100

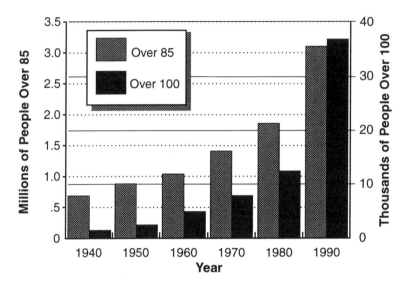

A third indicator of rising longevity is the astounding rise in the number of people living past 100. Before 1950, it was rare for anyone to live that long. In 1950, only 2,500 Americans were over 100. By 1980, the number was 12,500. Then, in a single decade, the number leaped to 37,000 by 1990. In the next four years, it rocketed to an estimated 51,000. By 2000, the United States Census Bureau estimates the number of Americans living past 100 will reach toward 100,000. The upward trend should continue. At this rate, there may be 200,000 people over 100 by 2010, and a million by 2030.

A fourth indicator of today's rising longevity is the increase in the maximum life span, the longest anyone has lived. Reports of long life have been with us since Biblical times. According to the Bible, Methuselah, son of Enoch and grandfather of Noah, lived 969 years. Adam and many generations of his descendants all lived more than 900 years. Then the longevity of succeeding generations de-

clined in a rather straight line, from 900 years downward to
around 500 years, then 200, then 70, and presumably on
down to the 20 years of Greek and Roman times.

There are claims of people living as long as 150 years
today in the Russian Caucasus, Vilcabamba in Ecuador, and
Hunza in the Kashmir of Pakistan. Regrettably, scientists
can't verify them from birth records. For two centuries,
Pierre Joubert of Canada held the verified maximum life
span. He lived from 1701 to 1814, a span of 113 years.
Since the maximum life span stayed at 113 for so long,
many scientists regarded 113 as a limit we could never
pass. Never say never. In the 1980s, as more people lived
past 100, some began to live 114, 115, and 116 years, all
verified by official birth records. By 1996, many had lived
past 113. Since the 113-year limit is nonsense, who has
lived the longest? For years, the *Guiness Book of World
Records* said it was Shigechiyo Izumi of Asan, Japan, who
died in 1986 after living to a reported age of 120 years, 237
days. Recently, though, the honor was given to Jeanne
Louise Calment of France. On February 21, 1997, she
reached a verified age of 122 years, surpassing Japan's
Izumi. In his book, *We Live Too Short and Die Too Long,*
however, Dr. W. M.. Bortz of Stanford University Medical
School related the case of Arthur Reed of Oakland, California. Birth records reported his life span reached 124 years.
Whatever today's maximum, as more people live past 100,
many should move toward 120. Chapter 7, however, will
show 120-130 to be the likely upper limit until we control
aging.

A surprising result of rising longevity is the better health
and vigor of older adults. From a survey in *Our Aging
Society: Paradox and Promise,* A. Pifer and L. Bronte report,
"Most men and women over 65 today are vigorous, healthy,
mentally alert, and still young in outlook." This seems to be
due to progress against diseases, access to good health care
for persons over 65, and increased emphasis on health and

fitness. A survey of 90-year-olds found 95 percent did not smoke, 88 percent did not drink in excess, and 77 percent exercised. Only 8 percent of people over 65 are in nursing homes. Many are victims not of age but of ailments like stroke, arthritis, heart failure, and Alzheimer's disease. To reduce nursing home populations, we must conquer those and similar diseases. The stereotype of feebleness as a part of old age is wrong. Except for victims of diseases, growing numbers of people over age 85 lead active lives.

The Road Ahead

Healthy lifestyles and high-tech medicine are pushing the life expectancy of health-conscious people past 100. All evidence suggests these trends will continue.

Today's science and technology are like nothing before in history. Research is progressing at an astonishing pace. Advances in medicine are coming at a rate unimaginable 20

Figure 1-5. Reports of Biomedical Advances

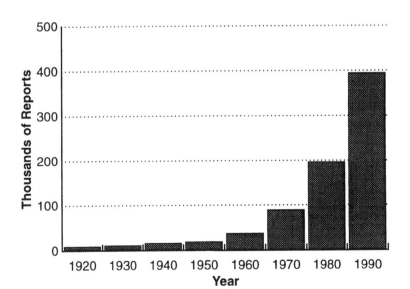

years ago. We see the dramatic change in Figure 1-5, which shows the thousands of reports of worldwide advances in research. They only began to rise in 1960 but have since skyrocketed. Dazzling progress is evident not only in medicine. In fact, advances in all sciences and technologies are so rapid today that it is difficult to keep up with them, even with the help of computerized databases. Advances that weren't expected, at best, for 20 or 30 years are appearing today. The National Library of Medicine is receiving 1,700 reports every day of new findings in biomedical research. Each year, research advances more rapidly. As a result of ever faster discovery, we have amassed a body of scientific and technological knowledge so vast that the human brain can't comprehend it without the aid of a computer. It is a base of immense power for further progress. Adding to our scientific and technological knowledge every week are a million scientists and engineers in thousands of laboratories around the world.

To further speed our progress, we have also witnessed an explosion of new techniques in science unequaled since the 1600s when modern science began. In the past, each jump forward in techniques set off a cascade of advances in knowledge. Today's explosion is likely to cause the biggest advances in history. During the next 20 years, we will extend life by continued progress against diseases, especially cardiovascular disease and cancer. By 2030 we should be able to prevent or cure 90 percent of today's ten leading causes of death. By 2050, another 20 years of progress should result in the conquest of most diseases. By 2080, after 30 additional years of progress, there should be few deaths from disease. Unthinkable? Just watch.

Aging will, however, initially limit our newfound longevity to 120 or 130 years. Thus, overcoming diseases will probably increase the numbers of 100- to 120-year-olds. Until now, aging has not been an immediate barrier to longer life because diseases usually kill us before aging has a chance. As we progress in the next 20 years against diseases, and health-conscious people live on past 85, aging will become a growing problem. Despite the amazing vigor of many persons older than 85, the ravages of aging will cause problems for those who may be free from many diseases but who will suffer the physical deterioration of the aging process. Fortunately, while the conquest of diseases occurs, we will extend today's progress against aging. If the current rate of advance continues, we should be able to slow human aging by 2030, possibly as early as 2015. This may affect you and many other persons alive today. We should be able to control aging by 2050 and virtually eliminate it, probably with gene therapy, by 2080.

Unthinkable? Splitting the atom was unthinkable in 1928, yet it occurred by 1938. Curing polio was inconceivable in 1949, but polio was almost wiped out by 1959. Travel to the moon seemed preposterous in 1954, yet it occurred in 1969. Genetic engineering was unimaginable in 1970, and it amazed us by 1980. There are hundreds of such examples. The control of aging is no more unthinkable than any of them.

How can you live longer? There are big signs pointing the way. Don't smoke. Exercise. Eat a balanced, low-fat diet high in fresh fruits and vegetables. Work closely with your physician to prevent and treat diseases. While doing these things, watch biomedical research conquer more diseases and move steadily toward the control of aging. A new era has arrived. We are off on the most exciting adventure that anyone, even Indiana Jones, could want—the journey toward long life.

2

The Conquest of Cardiovascular Disease

I am an out-and-out believer in preventive measures
against diseases as contrasted
with what are called curative agencies.
—Oliver Wendell Holmes, M.D.

We want to live longer, but the barrier of cardiovascular disease rears up before us like a great wall. It kills more of us than anything else, causing one of every three deaths. It stands in the same spot smallpox did for centuries prior to 1800. Before we can even think of stopping aging, we must first prevent cardiovascular disease. Happily, biomedical research is moving so rapidly that the barrier of cardiovascular disease is crumbling. Today, we can prevent or treat most of it. Preventive methods are appearing so fast that we haven't had enough time to measure their total effect. They may likely prevent 80 percent of cardiovascular disease. Cardiologists can treat much we don't prevent. As a result, health-conscious people have little cardiovascular disease. This contributes significantly to their 100-year lives. Still, many people fail to use available preventive measures. For them, cardiovascular disease is a big barrier to long life. They are the reason it is the leading cause of death.

Let's analyze the problem. Our circulatory system consists of the heart and blood vessels. The heart pumps oxygen-rich blood through arteries to the body's organs, including the heart. Veins carry carbon dioxide-rich blood back to the heart, which pumps it through the lungs to exchange carbon dioxide for oxygen. Oxygen-rich blood returns to the heart to be pumped again to the organs. The system works well, often for more than 100 years without repair. How many machines can do that? An engineer would recognize the problems that may occur in the cardiovascular system. They are the same as those of a pump and a network of pipes. Trouble comes when the pump or its controls don't work properly, or when the pipes clog or rupture. The root cause of most cardiovascular disease is clogged pipes!

Types of Cardiovascular Disease

To control cardiovascular disease, we first divide the problem into smaller, solvable ones, the way engineers subdivided the big problem of going to the moon. Figure 2-1 shows how cardiovascular disease splits nicely into five subproblems: atherosclerosis, heart attack, other ischemia, hypertension, and other heart diseases.

Atherosclerosis causes 70 percent of cardiovascular disease, including heart attacks, other ischemia, some hypertension, and some heart failure. It results when fatty materials (including cholesterol), cells, and proteins deposit on the inner walls of your blood vessels. As deposits build, the vessels narrow. This hinders blood flow, raises blood pressure, and triggers blood clots that can block a vessel completely. In the early stages, atherosclerosis has no obvious symptoms. As it develops, it causes pain. By that time, it needs urgent treatment, often with angioplasty or bypass surgery. These only treat its effects, not the disease itself, but they can save your life. In balloon angioplasty, a cardiologist runs a tube through blood vessels to a sector nar-

Figure 2-1. Cardiovascular Disease

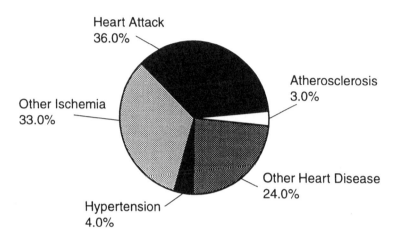

Heart Attack
36.0%

Atherosclerosis
3.0%

Other Ischemia
33.0%

Other Heart Disease
24.0%

Hypertension
4.0%

rowed by atherosclerosis and then inflates a balloon at the
end of the tube. This squeezes the deposits against the
walls, opening the vessel. It's imperfect treatment because
the effect is often temporary. It frequently damages the
walls of the blood vessels, causing a growth of cells that
narrows the vessel again. Still, it removes a blockage until
a better but slower treatment can cure atherosclerosis.
Coronary bypass surgery replaces a blocked artery with a
section of a vein from the leg. It, too, treats the effects of
atherosclerosis rather than the disease. Without preventative measures the new section of artery will clog again, but
this surgery is vital when a blockage is life threatening.

If your physician detects atherosclerosis early, less painful, less expensive, and more effective cures are at hand.
Dr. Dean Ornish, a physician and advocate of healthy lifestyles, has found that not smoking, exercise, and a low-fat
diet can remove 6-9 percent of atherosclerotic deposits.
These preventative measures didn't entirely eliminate
blockages but were safe and reduced deposits everywhere.
Most important, they show that deposits can be dissolved.

A more effective treatment adds cholesterol-lowering drugs to a healthy lifestyle. In one thirty-month study, researchers divided patients into three groups. Group A had only a low-fat diet and exercise. Group B also took the cholesterol-lowering drugs Colestid and Lovastatin. Group C also took Colestid, plus the B-vitamin niacin. The results? For group A, arteries opened in 11 percent of the patients, but 19 percent died of heart attacks. For group B, arteries opened in 32 percent of the patients, and only 7 percent died of heart attacks. For group C, arteries opened in 39 percent of the patients, and incredibly only 4 percent died of heart attacks. The drugs even stop atherosclerosis in familial hypercholesterolemia, a hereditary disease that often causes fatal atherosclerosis. In patients with this disease, a control group had a low-fat diet while a test group got Colestid or Lovastatin. The cholesterol level in the control group fell, but atherosclerosis increased. The test group not only had lower cholesterol levels, but atherosclerosis also declined. Recent studies have found that newer cholesterol-lowering drugs are even more effective. Their ability to treat atherosclerosis has enormous potential to conquer this disease.

A *heart attack* occurs when a blood clot plugs an artery supplying your heart. The artery is usually already narrowed by atherosclerosis. The clot stops the blood supply to part of the heart. Heart attacks hit abruptly and often fatally. On average, 25 percent of victims die instantly. Fifty percent die within hours or days. Twenty-five percent recover, with some heart damage. Symptoms of a heart attack include gripping pain in the chest, shortness of breath, a feeling of apprehension, clammy skin, and sometimes nausea. Quick action in getting to a hospital emergency room is vital. Cardiologists prefer to respond to a false alarm than to take a chance on the real thing. Treatment with aspirin, heparin, or a thrombolytic (clot-dissolving) enzyme like TPA or streptokinase sharply reduces heart attack deaths. In

17,000 heart attacks, streptokinase plus aspirin lowered deaths 50 percent. TPA with aspirin and heparin reduced deaths among 700 heart attack patients 40 percent. *Other ischemia* occurs when arteries, gradually closed by atherosclerosis, cut off oxygen to your heart or other organs. In arteries supplying your heart, it causes the clutching pain of angina in the chest and the fatal deterioration of heart action. Narrowed arteries feeding leg muscles cause the pain of claudication. Narrowed arteries feeding the brain cause stroke-like symptoms and the dizziness of transient ischemic attacks. Narrowed arteries feeding your kidneys cause their failure. Although most ischemia results from atherosclerosis, it is also caused by injury to an artery, the spasm of a wall muscle in an artery, or inadequate blood flow due to inefficient heart pumping. The pain of ischemia may be eased by drugs. A cure, however, requires not smoking, a healthy diet, exercise, and cholesterol-lowering drugs. In acute cases, angioplasty or surgery may be necessary.

Hypertension occurs when blood pressure is consistently above 140/90. It leads to stroke, heart failure, kidney damage, injury to the retinas, confusion, and death. Causes are atherosclerosis, smoking, constricted blood vessels, poor kidney function, lead in your environment, and heavily salted food. One of every four adults in the United States suffers from high blood pressure, but an astounding two-thirds do nothing about it until it's too late. The incidence of hypertension is similar in many nations. An array of drugs can treat hypertension. Diuretics lower blood pressure by reducing salt and water. Calcium channel blockers relax blood vessel walls. Beta blockers slow the heart rate and curb a protein that raises blood pressure. ACE inhibitors stop the constriction of arteries. The drugs don't cure the problem, but they usually lower blood pressure to a safe level.

Other heart diseases include injury, infection, arrhythmia, heart block, heart failure, cardiomyopathy, and birth defects. *Injury* often occurs in auto accidents when the steering wheel rams the heart, or from drugs. *Infection* occurs when bacteria in the blood attack the heart, as in rheumatic fever, illegal drug use, or surgery. *Arrhythmia* and *heart block* are defects in heartbeat. *Heart failure* is the inability of the heart to keep up its workload. *Cardiomyopathy* is a deterioration of the heart muscle. Together, they cause only a fourth of cardiovascular disease, so each affects a relatively small percentage of people.

Surgery can treat both injury and birth defects, antibiotics can treat infection, and drugs or a pacemaker implant can treat arrhythmia. Symptoms of heart failure are fatigue, breathlessness (especially after exertion), and swelling of the ankles or legs. These symptoms are often eased by diuretic drugs to remove extra fluid, vasodilators to ease the heart's work, and digitalis to strengthen the heartbeat. The drug vesnarinone slows the deterioration of heart function and cuts deaths from heart failure in half. ACE inhibitors strikingly reduce heart failure.

Some cardiomyopathy results from heavy drinking, but the cause of most cases remains unknown. The combined drugs hydralazine and isosorbide dinitrate lower deaths by 21 percent, and enalapril drops deaths by 35 percent. For years, a heart transplant was the only cure for cardiomyopathy. Although transplants are increasingly successful, there aren't enough hearts to fill the need. Now, growth hormones have shown a remarkable ability to restore much of a heart damaged by cardiomyopathy. This exciting finding indicates we may soon enter an era when physicians can restore many hearts without transplants.

Prevention of Cardiovascular Disease

The best way to defeat cardiovascular disease is to prevent it. It is always easier to prevent a disease than to cure it. You can extend your life to an astounding degree with simple acts of prevention. Biomedical research finds more cures each year, but preventive medicine is our future. It extends life by promoting a healthy lifestyle, immunization, and accident reduction. Its ability against infectious disease is legendary. It has wiped smallpox from the earth, is ridding us of polio, and it is doing the same for cardiovascular disease. The actions you can take to prevent most cardiovascular disease are familiar but amazingly effective.

Don't Smoke

Not smoking will prevent more cardiovascular disease than anything else. Everyone knows smoking is deadly. It is the main cause of preventable deaths in the United States, killing more than 400,000 people per year. It annually kills more Americans than World War I, the Korean War, and the Vietnam War combined did, and almost as many as World War II did. Massive evidence reported by the U.S. Surgeon General leaves no doubt that smoking is the nation's leading killer.

Smoking is also the chief source of cardiovascular disease, causing half its deaths. The evidence for this is enormous, but look at just one example. Figure 2-2 shows findings on more than 100,000 women by Dr. Walter Willett and his coworkers at the Harvard School of Public Health. They found that the risk of dying from cardiovascular disease rises with the number of cigarettes smoked per day. Someone who smokes a pack per day has almost four times the risk of a nonsmoker. Someone who smokes more than two packs per day has ten times the risk. But this cloud has a silver lining. Figure 2-2 shows that when people quit smoking, the risk drops to only slightly more than that of nonsmokers within two years. This greater *risk of dying* of cardiovascular disease translates into smokers *actually dying* twice as fast from it and from all other causes. Non-

Figure 2-2. Smoking and Heart Disease

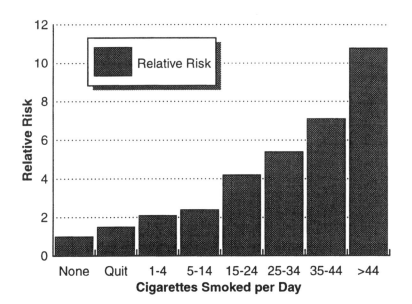

Cigarettes Smoked per Day

smokers have far fewer deaths from cardiovascular disease. For example, Dr. James Enstrom of UCLA measured cardiovascular disease deaths in nearly 10,000 Mormons, ages 25-99, who don't smoke for religious reasons. They had half the deaths as occur generally. This statistic is not unique to Mormons. Enstrom found that 2,000 non-Mormon nonsmokers also had half the deaths from cardiovascular disease. Other researchers have found the same thing.

This tells us something important. If no one smoked, deaths from cardiovascular disease would be only half of what they are. Not smoking can do more to reduce cardiovascular disease than any cures. It extends your life expectancy a surprising amount and is the first step toward long life.

Exercise

Nonsmokers can lower cardiovascular disease further with moderate exercise, such as a daily 30 to 45 minute walk. For nonsmokers, such exercise reduces deaths from cardiovascular disease an additional 10 percent. That doesn't seem like much, but together with not smoking, it cuts your chance of dying from cardiovascular disease by 60 percent. Instead of 10 percent, you can cut it 14 percent by walking five miles per week and 16 percent by walking ten miles.

Adequate Sleep

Seven to eight hours of sleep per night by exercising non-smokers lowers cardiovascular disease deaths an additional 6 percent.

Figure 2-3 shows the astonishing drop in deaths from cardiovascular disease caused by these three preventative actions. Not smoking, moderate exercise, and adequate sleep can prevent almost two-thirds of deaths from cardiovascular disease.

There are other ways for you to further prevent cardiovascular disease. In fact, preventive methods are coming faster than researchers can measure their effects on exercising nonsmokers.

Optimal Weight

In nonsmokers, the correct body weight helps prevent more cardiovascular disease. If you keep your weight in the desirable range, it does three things for you. It prevents obesity, a killer. It extends life. It helps keep your cholesterol level in the healthy range, preventing atherosclerosis.

You are *obese* if you weigh 20 percent more than the desirable weight for your height. The average weights of Americans have climbed eight pounds in the past 15 years, so more people are obese. Table 2-1 shows examples of obesity for men and women.

Figure 2-3. Prevention of Cardiovascular Disease

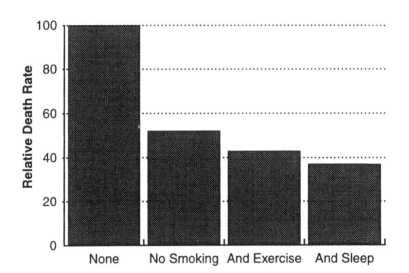

Obesity more than doubles the risk of dying of cardio-vascular disease. In 1995, 40 percent of U.S. adults were obese, up from 33 percent in 1990 and 25 percent in 1980. Half of young people under 18 are grossly overweight, and their gain is out of control. Being overweight, but not obese, still raises the risk of dying. Women averaging 158 pounds have 1.5 times the risk of dying of a heart attack as women at 118 pounds, while those averaging 192 pounds have more than twice the risk. Dr. Joann Manson and her colleagues at Harvard found that nonsmokers further re-

Table 2-1

Men			Women		
Height	Desirable Weight	Obese	Height	Desirable Weight	Obese
5'2"	129 lbs	155 lbs	5'1"	112 lbs	134 lbs
5'7"	147 lbs	177 lbs	5'6"	129 lbs	155 lbs
6'0"	167 lbs	201 lbs	6'0"	152 lbs	182 lbs

duce cardiovascular disease deaths as they lower their weight to the desirable level. Even small decreases in weight reduce the risk proportionately. Very thin persons, weighing less than the desirable level, often have a higher mortality rate than those in the desirable weight range. This is due to smoking or disease among those individuals. For healthy, exercising, nonsmokers the thinner we are, the longer we live.

To control weight, we can't avoid the basic equation: calories in = calories out. To maintain a healthy weight, you must balance food intake against exercise. If you eat more calories than you use, you gain weight. If you eat fewer calories than you use, you lose weight. You attain the desirable weight by combined diet and exercise. To do it, you must not starve yourself. Instead, you reduce calories in by eating all you want of no-calorie or low-calorie foods. If necessary, you might also take anti-obesity drugs such as fenfluramine or phentermine. You increase calories out by increasing your exercise, especially walking. This combination maintains weight loss, while merely starving on a diet does not. A study of 288 people who have lived past 100 found almost all were in the desirable weight range. They also reported that they exercised (by working) throughout their lives.

Healthy Diet

Constantly eating more calories than you use is likely to cause atherosclerosis. Your excess calories convert to fatty matter, especially cholesterol, which deposits on and narrows the walls of your arteries. A blood cholesterol level of less than 200 milligrams per deciliter (mg/dl) is ideal, 201-240 mg/dl is risky, and above 240 mg/dl is bad. Figure 2-4 shows how deaths from cardiovascular disease rise with blood cholesterol level. Deaths increase significantly when the blood cholesterol level is above 200. People with a level of 264 have almost five times the deaths of those with

Figure 2-4. Cholesterol and Heart Disease

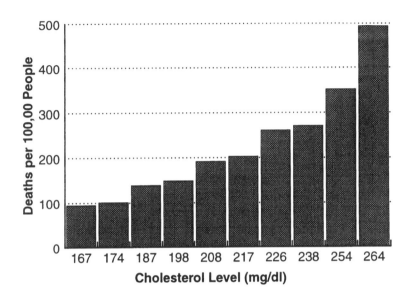

a level of 198. Replacing fats with reasonable amounts of carbohydrates and proteins stops atherosclerosis. We see it if we substitute rice (90 percent carbohydrates and 10 percent proteins) for fats. The Chinese, who eat a lot of rice and little fat, have cholesterol levels averaging 127, compared to 212 in the United States. The Japanese, also rice eaters with low cholesterol levels, have a life expectancy 4 years longer than Americans.

Cholesterol-Lowering Drugs

If diet can't get your cholesterol down, drugs can. Combined with a low-fat diet, they stop atherosclerosis. A study of more than 8,000 patients with high cholesterol found the drug Lovastatin lowered levels 24-40 percent. A low dosage lowers a blood cholesterol level of 250 to 190, while a high dosage reduces a level of 300 to 180. A five-year study of the drug Simvastatin on 4,400 patients revealed that it reduces heart attack deaths more than 40 percent, nonfatal heart attacks 30 percent, and bypass surgery 37 percent. Cholesterol-lowering drugs have enormous potential to prevent atherosclerosis. Combined with not smoking, exercise, and desirable weight, they give us the ability to prevent 70 percent of cardiovascular disease.

Aspirin

Heart attacks are dangerous because they kill instantly in 25 percent of all cases. Prevention is essential. Recall that almost all heart attacks occur when atherosclerosis narrows a coronary artery, and a blood clot plugs the artery at the narrow spot. One 2.5-grain aspirin tablet per day greatly reduces the formation of clots. Dr. Manson's team found aspirin lowers the risk of heart attack 32 percent in women and 44 percent in men. We now need to know how much additional reduction in cardiovascular disease occurs when exercising nonsmokers take a daily aspirin.

Annual Medical Exam

Cardiovascular disease is easier to cure if found early. Blood pressure, cholesterol and lipoprotein levels, electrocardiograms, and other diagnostic tools can detect it at an early stage when treatment is most effective. A thorough exam by your physician is essential every year.

Prevent Hypertension

Since the causes of hypertension are atherosclerosis, smoking, obesity, stress, lead, salt, diabetes, and alcohol, the best way to prevent it is to avoid these hazards. Sadly, many hypertensives are obese fat-eaters who smoke, drink, and salt their food heavily.

Estrogen Use by Postmenopausal Women

Early in life, women have far less cardiovascular disease than men. After menopause, their rate jumps to equal that of men. Low doses of estrogen cut cardiovascular disease almost in half. It will be fascinating to see the effect of estrogen on cardiovascular disease in nonsmoking women who exercise and maintain a desirable weight. They likely will have almost no cardiovascular disease.

Exercising nonsmokers already avoid almost two-thirds of cardiovascular disease. Desirable weight, low cholesterol, a daily aspirin, regular medical exams, and estrogen for postmenopausal women will also help prevent cardiovascular disease. Researchers have not had enough time to determine the total effect of these measures. If they reduce deaths only 3 percent each, they would together prevent almost 80 percent of cardiovascular disease. In his book, *Rx 2000*, on the future of medicine and health, Dr. Jeffrey Fisher predicts better prevention and treatment will eliminate the need for 75 percent of bypass surgery in the year 2000, and 95 percent by 2011.

It is more difficult, however, to prevent the remaining 20 percent of cardiovascular disease. We must deter injury, infection, damage, arrhythmia, and heart failure. We can prevent many heart injuries by redesigning the steering wheels in motor vehicles. Minimal use of damaging drugs will prevent still more injuries. Antibiotic therapy now used before surgery prevents many infections of the heart. We can prevent some heart failure by not smoking, controlling blood pressure, repairing deficient heart valves, and by preventing anemia, hyperthyroidism, and heart attack. Indeed, we may already be able to prevent more than 80 percent of cardiovascular disease.

Experimental Advances in Prevention and Treatment

Research is progressing to find even more ways to prevent or treat atherosclerosis, hypertension, heart attacks, heart failure, and other heart diseases. Let's look at a few.

Vitamin E

Analysis of sixteen populations in Europe found that people with cardiovascular disease also have low levels of vitamin E. Those with high levels of vitamin E have less. In fact, the level of vitamin E is a better predictor of cardiovascular disease than either cholesterol level or blood pressure. This suggests vitamin E may help prevent cardiovascular disease. Evidence comes from several large studies. Among 87,000 women, those who took at least 100 units of vitamin E per day had 41 percent less cardiovascular disease. A study of almost 40,000 men found that nonsmokers who took at least 100 units of vitamin E per day had a similar drop in cardiovascular disease, but it was not as effective for smokers. Spectacular results came from feeding 2,000 people, all prone to heart attacks, a daily 800 units of vitamin E. It caused a 75 percent drop in deaths from cardiovascular disease.

Vitamin C

A study of 11,000 adults found that 500 milligrams of vitamin C per day lowers cardiovascular disease deaths 42 percent in men and 25 percent in women. Another study found that combining vitamin C and vitamin E causes a 50 percent drop in cardiovascular disease.

Anti-Obesity Protein

Researchers have found in mice a gene they named *obese,* because damage to it causes mice to become hugely fat. A similar gene is in humans. It's the pattern for a protein, leptin, which controls weight. If you inject leptin into obese mice, they revert to normal. Researchers want to know whether we can control human obesity with similar proteins or drugs.

Hundreds of new drugs and methods to treat cardiovascular disease appear every year. Researchers are testing the replacement of angioplasty balloons with high-speed grinders and lasers. After angioplasty, they are using tubular inserts in arteries to stop further narrowing. Cholesterol-lowering drugs are increasingly able to wipe out atherosclerosis. Research is also moving against familial hypercholesterolemia, the hereditary disease that kills by atherosclerosis. Researchers have inserted a cholesterol-destroying gene into the liver cells of rabbits. When injected back into the rabbits, the liver cells lower cholesterol levels 30 percent. Much work remains before use in humans, but gene therapy may overcome this disease. Researchers are finding faster ways to diagnose heart attacks, but a major problem for survivors is damage to the heart. Researchers have found that the drug TGF-B given to animals soon after an attack, cuts damage in half. Basic FGF, another drug, causes new blood vessels to grow into a damaged heart, reducing dead muscle and improving heart function.

Drop In Deaths From Cardiovascular Disease

Even though many persons still kill themselves with smoking, high-fat diets, and no exercise, Figure 2-5 shows that prevention and treatment are reducing deaths. In 1950, deaths began to decline. By 1990, they had fallen 31 percent and are still dropping. If current progress continues, Figure 2-5 projects deaths at half the 1950 rate by the year 2000, at 30 percent of that rate by 2010, and almost gone by 2030. This is similar to a forecast by Dr. Fisher in *Rx 2000*, based on interviews with medical researchers. He predicts deaths from cardiovascular disease will drop 85 percent by 2010 and 99 percent by 2030. If these projections are nearly correct, cardiovascular disease will no longer be a big killer by 2010 and almost vanish by 2030. Nobel laureates Michael Brown and Joseph Goldstein also predict an end to cardiovascular disease as a major problem early in the twenty-first century. Evidence that all these forecasts are correct appears almost faster than we can grasp it. Our knowledge of atherosclerosis is exploding.

Figure 2-5. Drop in Cardiovascular Disease

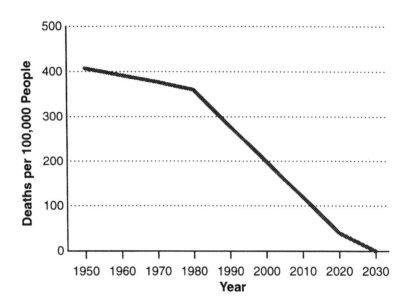

Ever better drugs are wiping out this cause of 70 percent of cardiovascular disease.

It doesn't stop there. Of the remaining 30 percent of cardiovascular disease, the big fraction caused by heart failure is falling to new drugs and to left-ventricular-assist devices. These can boost failing hearts so much that patients can live normal lives. Another big part of that 30 percent, arrhythmia, is yielding to implanted defibrillators that sense trouble and shock the heart into a normal rhythm. As researchers identify genes for cardiomyopathies, arrhythmia, and less-known diseases, therapies will follow. The pace of discovery is so fast that our ability to eliminate almost all cardiovascular disease by 2030 may be a conservative projection. It likely will come sooner.

Rise in Life Expectancy from Progress Against Cardiovascular Disease

How much does our ability to prevent and treat cardiovascular disease raise life expectancy? As deaths drop in a population, life expectancy rises. Anything that lowers deaths raises life expectancy. We may calculate life expectancy from life tables provided by the National Center for Health Statistics. These tables show how many persons of each age die per 100,000 people in a particular year. If you are curious about calculating life expectancy, Marion Lamb's *Biology of Aging* offers a clear explanation. The equations may appear formidable, but life expectancy may be calculated in the blink of an eye by computer.

Recall that the life expectancy of newborns in the United States is 76 years. Adults can expect to live longer. Remember, the longer you have lived, the longer you can expect to live.

■ Life expectancy at birth = 76 years.

■ Life expectancy at age 35 = 78 years.

■ Life expectancy at age 65 = 82 years.

Now, let's see how preventative actions against cardiovascular disease raise life expectancy. Nonsmokers have 48 percent fewer deaths from cardiovascular disease. The drop in deaths from not smoking adds 6 years to your life.

■ Life expectancy of non-smokers at age 35 = 84 years.

■ Life expectancy of non-smokers at age 65 = 88 years.

Since growing numbers of people don't smoke, it is no wonder that people living past 85 are increasing six times faster than any other age group. That's not all. Nonsmokers who exercise regularly and get adequate sleep have 63 percent fewer deaths from cardiovascular disease.

■ Life expectancy of exercising non-smokers at age 35 = 86 years.

- Life expectancy of exercising non-smokers at age 65
  = 90 years.

Desirable weight, a proper diet, medical exams, aspirin, cholesterol-lowering drugs, and estrogen for post-menopausal women also reduce cardiovascular disease. Vitamins E and C may also be beneficial. We don't yet know how much all these preventive measures lower deaths in nonsmokers who exercise. But if they lower deaths by an average of only 3 percent each, they can raise prevention to at least 75 percent.

- Life expectancy of health-conscious people at age 35
  = 87 years.
- Life expectancy of health-conscious people at age 65
  = 91 years.

Thus, our ability to prevent cardiovascular disease today can extend your life 9 years. Future advances will raise life expectancy further. The added years will likely be healthy ones. A study of old adults by the National Institute on Aging found that the most active adults do not smoke, have normal weight, and suffer from neither hypertension nor arthritis.

The Road Ahead

For years, cardiovascular disease has stood as the first barrier to longer life. Now, research has made so much progress that we can prevent or cure 70-80 percent. The only thing that allows cardiovascular disease to continue as a barrier is the large number of people who fail to take these simple actions to prevent it.

- Don't smoke
- Exercise moderately.
- Get 7-8 hours of sleep.
- Eat a balanced, low-fat diet.
- Maintain optimal weight.
- Take a 2.5-grain aspirin tablet daily.

- Have a medical exam yearly.
- Consider cholesterol-lowering drugs.
- Postmenopausal women should take estrogen.

At the same time, research continues on ways to prevent or treat the remainder of cardiovascular disease. All evidence is that rapid progress will continue to move toward the seemingly inconceivable—the conquest of all cardiovascular disease. The continuation of current progress will soon yield new drugs that are more effective at preventing atherosclerosis. For treatment, better cholesterol-lowering drugs will be more effective at reducing atherosclerotic deposits. By the year 2010, specific solubilizing agents or enzymes will remove deposits completely. This will wipe out most heart attacks, other angina, and much of the cardiovascular disease that we have not already prevented. Continued research will soon develop stronger thrombolytic and support drugs to treat the heart attacks we don't prevent. Tests will predict the likelihood of a heart attack. Home kits will diagnose a heart attack and provide support medication until help arrives. Drugs will restore damaged heart muscle to normal. Other heart diseases will be the last to disappear. Continued research will move toward cures with gene therapy to repair congenital heart defects, drugs to reverse heart failure, and either gene therapy or drugs to reverse the deterioration of heart muscle in cardiomyopathy.

The extension of today's progress will provide ever better prevention and treatment of cardiovascular disease. By the year 2030, cardiovascular disease should almost disappear among health-conscious people. How quickly it vanishes will depend on how well the population becomes health conscious. If enough people do, cardiovascular disease could be nothing but a memory in the twenty-first century.

This first step to living longer can raise your life expectancy to 86 or 87 years. To raise your life expectancy higher, we must overcome cancer. Next, we will view that barrier and see how we can dismantle it to extend life further.

3

Progress Against Cancer

The golden age of medicine is at hand
—Dr. George Lundberg

You triumphantly surmount the barrier of cardiovascular disease and look ahead to 87 years of healthy life. Beyond 87, blocking progress to 100, sits the barrier of cancer. Cancer causes one-fourth of all deaths. The disease is so daunting that people often regard a diagnosis of cancer as a death sentence. It isn't, but progress against cancer has been slow. In past years, you may have heard a cure was "just around the corner," but it wasn't.

Today, the outlook is brighter because of rapid advances in medicine. In fact, Dr. George Lundberg, editor of the *Journal of the American Medical Association* has said, "In developed countries, the golden age of medicine is at hand—for the patients." He cites advances in science, abundant technology, excellent facilities, enough physicians, fast communication, preventive medicine, and scientific management as bases for his view. The golden age includes progress against cancer based on molecular biology, immunology, and genetic engineering.

What Is Cancer?

Let's begin again by analyzing the problem. Cancer is an abnormal growth of cells in the body. It is parasitic and causes toxemia, a generalized poisoning. As the growth advances, it becomes *malignant.* Cells slough off the cancer and travel throughout the body to form new masses. Left alone, the original cell mass or one of the new masses will grow until it stops a vital function, killing you.

Hence, the problem we face with cancer is different from the trouble with the "pump" or "clogged pipes" of cardiovascular disease. Cancer results from damage to key genes in our DNA, a long thread in our cells. DNA is composed of thousands of genes that control every facet of life. DNA is like a videotape that plays a series of scenes showing you how to do different things. Instead of instructional scenes, DNA has genes. The genes tell your cells how to produce and operate the thousands of parts of your body. There are also genes that control other genes. At any moment, control genes can "switch on" thousands of genes to keep us operating properly or "switch off" thousands more until needed.

You grow when a set of *growth genes* switches on. When you reach the proper size, the growth genes switch off. To be certain you stop growing, a set of *tumor suppressor genes* switches on as a backup system in case the growth genes fail to switch off. This keeps your cells from growing wildly to a point where the mass of cells would kill you. The problem is that environmental hazards such as radiation or chemicals can damage your genes. Most damage has little effect because your cells have an efficient system to repair your DNA. But on rare occasions, damage causes a growth gene to switch on permanently or disables a tumor suppressor gene. As a result, a cell may become precancerous. It's not a problem unless more damage later switches on other growth genes and disables other tumor suppressor genes. Then you have cancer.

The bad news about cancer is that it will kill you if you don't act against it. The good news is that it requires damage to an *entire series of genes* before a cell becomes cancerous. It takes repeated, long-term exposure to radiation or chemicals (cigarette smoke, for example) to damage the series of genes. Thus, if we know what causes each kind of cancer, prevention is possible by avoiding the cause.

Since cancer results from damage to genes, a cure is difficult because we do not have an easy way to repair damaged genes. We likely will be able to repair them in the future. Today, prevention of damage is easier than a cure.

Cancer is not a single disease. Liver cancers differ from lung cancers, which differ from colon cancers. Some grow slowly, while others grow with amazing speed. Cancers also differ in how frequently each kind occurs and how often they kill people. Figure 3-1 shows the leading killers. In women, lung and breast cancers are tops. Each causes about one of every five cancer deaths. Colon cancer is close behind, then cancers of the pancreas and ovary. To-

Figure 3-1. Most Frequent Cancers

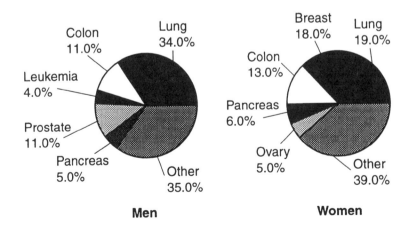

Men   Women

gether, the five cause 61 percent of all cancer deaths in women. In men, lung cancer is the big killer, causing one of every three cancer deaths. Colon and prostate cancers follow, then pancreatic cancer and leukemia. Together, the five cause 65 percent of all cancer deaths in men. Other cancers kill fewer people. They range from skin cancer (especially malignant melanoma), which kills 3 percent, down to cancers that kill a fraction of 1 percent. That lesser-occurring cancers together kill 35 percent shows they can form in almost any tissue.

Prevention Of Cancer

We can divide the large problem of cancer prevention into the subproblems of preventing each kind. Different agents damage DNA and cause different cancers. Smoking causes the biggest killer, lung cancer, but we do not know the causes of many cancers. Below are the known and possible causes of cancers, in order of how often each cancer occurs. The list is from the review "Toward the Primary Prevention of Cancer."

Cancer	Known or Possible Causes
Lung	Smoking
Colon/rectum	Fat, low fiber, alcohol, sedentary life
Breast	Ovarian hormones
Prostate	Testosterone, estrogen
Uterus	Estrogen
Mouth/throat	Smoking, alcohol
Pancreas	Smoking
Leukemia	X rays
Melanoma	Ultraviolet light
Kidney	Smoking, analgesics, diuretics
Stomach	Smoking, salt, Helicobacter pylori
Brain	Trauma, X rays

This collection of more than 100 research reports by Drs. B.E. Henderson, R.K. Ross, and M.C. Pike of the University of Southern California, appeared in the journal *Science*. In it, you will see that smoking is the most frequent cause of cancer. Fat, hormones, radiation, alcohol, salt, and even a stomach bacterium also cause cancers. There are surely other causes. We do not know as many ways to prevent cancer as we do to prevent cardiovascular disease. This explains why cardiovascular disease is dropping so much faster than cancer. Still, the preventive methods we have are effective.

Don't Smoke

Smoking is the killer again here. Smoking causes one-third of all cancer deaths, so a nonsmoker has a far lesser chance of getting cancer. Smoking causes almost all lung cancer, cancer of the larynx, cancer of the mouth, plus most cancer of the esophagus. It causes almost half of bladder cancer, a fourth of colon cancer, and some cancer of the stomach and pancreas. Although it doesn't cause all cancers (breast and prostate cancers, for example), smoking is responsible for an appalling amount of cancer. The need for prevention is clear. In a study of almost 10,000 nonsmokers, Dr. James Enstrom of UCLA found that not smoking cuts deaths from cancer almost in half. Not smoking wipes out three-fourths of deaths from all smoking-related cancers.

Nonsmokers have almost no lung cancer. Nonsmokers tend to avoid smokers and places where smoking is permitted. The virtual absence of lung cancer in nonsmokers may not only be the product of not smoking but also of not breathing secondhand smoke. Smokers put nonsmokers, including children, at risk of dying. Harvard School of Public Health researchers have studied the lungs of smokers, nonsmokers, and nonsmokers married to smokers. In contrast to the clean lungs of nonsmokers, smokers have many precancerous lesions in their lungs. But the most startling finding was that nonsmokers married to smokers also have many precancerous lesions. At least 50,000 nonsmokers die each year from breathing secondhand smoke. The hazard is so bad that the U.S. Environmental Protection Agency has declared tobacco smoke in closed areas to be a carcinogen. The agency has urged a ban on smoking in public places.

Not smoking cuts total deaths from cancer almost in half and nearly wipes out lung cancer. No other action you can take is as effective in preventing cancer.

Low-Fat Diet

Increased body weight above the desirable level causes a rise in deaths primarily from breast, colon, endometrial, prostate, and pancreatic cancer. Dr. Walter Willett and his associates at Harvard have found women's risk of colon cancer to be almost twice as high for those who eat the most fat compared with those who eat the least. Figure 3-2 compares colon cancer among the Chinese on their low-fat diet with colon cancer among Americans (including Chinese-Americans) on their high-fat diet. By age 65, Americans have three times the colon cancer of the Chinese, and by age 85, nine times more. Americans, who get 45 percent of their calories from fat, have high death rates from breast, colon, prostate, ovary, endometrium, and pancreatic cancer. The Japanese, who get 15 percent of their calories from fat, have far fewer deaths from these cancers. Instead, the Japanese have more stomach cancer from eating heavily salted food. Researchers have found that prostate cancer grows less than half as fast on a diet containing 21 percent fat compared with a diet of 40 percent fat, the level often eaten by American men. Since prostate cancer is so widespread in older men, a low-fat diet could slow cancer growth until an effective treatment appears.

Figure 3-2. Diet and Colon Cancer

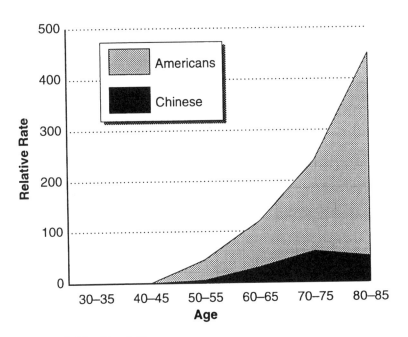

Annual Medical Exam

Essential for the prevention of cancer deaths is early detection, when treatment is most likely to succeed. Medical exams can often do this, especially for the leading hazards: lung, colon, breast, and prostate cancer.

Lung Cancer

Regular chest X rays usually detect it. Prevention (not smoking and avoiding secondhand smoke) and early detection can wipe out almost all deaths.

Colon Cancer

An occult blood test each year and a sigmoidoscopy every 3-5 years can provide early detection. Sigmoidoscopy is a painless procedure in which a physician inserts a flexible tube through the rectum to view the lower colon. A regular sigmoidoscopy for patients in the Kaiser Medical Program cut the risk of dying from colon cancer 60-70 percent. The American Cancer Society reports early detection results in 92 percent survival.

Breast Cancer

A breast self-examination monthly and a periodic mammography detects it at a treatable stage. For women over 50, mammography should be yearly. Early detection should require only minimal surgery and result in 97 percent survival.

Prostate Cancer

Approximately 80 percent of men over 80 develop prostate cancer. Although it often grows slowly, monitoring is vital. The prostate-specific antigen (PSA) test is a sensitive detector of prostate cancer. The more advanced the cancer, the higher the PSA level. The normal range is 1-4; a 10 needs investigation. A yearly PSA test combined with a digital exam increases accuracy. Early detection results in 99 percent survival.

Thorough medical examinations are powerful preventive methods. They detect many cancers in the earliest stages, when cures are most successful.

Aspirin

In a study of more than 660,000 persons, researchers for the American Cancer Society found those who took an aspirin every other day had only 60 percent as many deaths from colon cancer. Acetaminophen (Tylenol, for example) had no effect.

Avoid Excess Iron

An important advance toward the prevention of colon cancer was the discovery that excess iron is a cause of colon cancer in men and postmenopausal women. Iron is linked with health, so an excess often comes from the use of multivitamins, which have 5-27 milligrams per tablet.

The recommended daily allowance is 18 mg, and you may get that much from food. Men and postmenopausal women can help prevent iron-induced colon cancer by using a multivitamin having 0-5 milligrams of iron. Donating blood to a local blood bank is a good way to rid yourself of excess iron.

Protection From Sunlight

Skin cancer, mostly from sunlight, causes 3 percent of all cancer deaths. Sunscreen or protective clothing is essential as the ozone layer degrades. Soaring cases of skin cancer (including malignant melanoma) mean that many persons aren't protecting themselves.

Experimental Advances in Prevention

Ongoing research is searching for ways to prevent even more cancer. Many preventive methods are still under study in the laboratory, but some have progressed to tests in humans.

Vitamin E

In the laboratory, large doses of vitamin E prevent almost all colon cancer in rats given dimethylhydrazine, a powerful cancer inducer. Many researchers have confirmed that vitamin E inhibits cancer. In 60,000 people, researchers found that the higher the vitamin E level in blood, the less cancer occurred. In a study of 35,000 women, those taking vitamin E had a 68 percent lower risk of colon cancer. In another study, vitamin E cut in half the risk of mouth or throat cancer. It appears that a 400-unit capsule of vitamin E is an effective aid in preventing several, possibly many, kinds of cancer. More studies to confirm this are in progress.

Selenium

Except in tiny amounts, selenium is poisonous. Some soils in the American West contain selenium. Plants absorb it. When cattle eat the plants, selenium causes a fatal disease called "staggers." In trace amounts, selenium is essential to us. It is part of a protein that helps protect our cells against damage from oxygen. Thus, we must have a little selenium in our diet. Selenium prevents a third of skin cancer and breast cancer in laboratory animals. Vitamin E has a strong ability to prevent colon cancer but little ability to prevent breast cancer. Together, selenium and vitamin E prevent more than half of breast cancer in animals. In a study of 3,000 persons, selenium in the diet cut in half the risk of lung cancer. In another study of 1,700 elderly persons, selenium cut sharply the occurrence of polyps, often precursors of cancer, in the colon. We need studies to determine whether a combination of selenium and vitamin E will prevent breast cancer in humans as it does in laboratory animals.

Beta-Carotene

Twenty studies have found that people with diets high in beta-carotene have less cancer than those with a lower intake. In more than 25,000 people, researchers found those with lung cancer had lower levels of beta-carotene and vitamin E than those without lung cancer. But beta-carotene doesn't prevent all cancers. High doses did not prevent skin cancer, for example.

Vitamin C

In human cells in the laboratory, vitamin C keeps cancer-causing chemicals from altering cells, making them cancerous. It has even caused cancer cells to revert to normal. Vitamin C inhibits stomach cancer. Forty-six studies of thousands of people show a high intake of vitamin C prevents half of oral, pancreas, lung, breast, and stomach cancer. In more than 11,000 people, 500 milligrams of vitamin C per day reduced cancer deaths 22 percent in men and 14 percent in women. Vitamin C has another role. When vitamin E inhibits cancer formation, the action inactivates vitamin E. Vitamin C changes vitamin E back to an active form, so it can continue to prevent cancer.

These substances are so promising that you may want to supplement your multivitamin with 400 units of vitamin E, 1,000 milligrams of vitamin C, 100 milligrams of selenium, and possibly beta-carotene. Researchers will soon know how much more cancer a combination of vitamin E, vitamin C, beta-carotene, and selenium prevents in nonsmokers. We must know optimal doses and whether they prevent others such as prostate, pancreatic, or ovarian cancer.

Treatment of Cancer

The best way to cure cancer is to get cell growth under control. Until we found what controls cell growth, we could not do this. Thus, cancers have been treated by removing them or killing them. *Surgery* simply cuts out the cancer. As long as the cancer cells have not spread, it has cured enormous numbers of cases. *Radiation* kills cancer cells. Radiologists focus radiation on cancer cells to minimize killing the surrounding normal cells. It is especially effective against cancers that have spread locally and are not readily treated by surgery. In some cases, combined surgery and radiation are more effective than either alone. The two main drawbacks of radiation are that it kills cells near the cancer and that it can cause radiation sickness. *Chemotherapy* stops cell growth, stopping cancer. Since most cells are not growing, it is somewhat specific. It succeeds more than people realize against leukemias and cancers that have spread. Combined chemotherapy and radiation may be more effective than chemotherapy alone. The major drawback of chemotherapy is that it acts against all growing cells. It prevents formation of blood cells, immune cells, and replacement cells as well. Chemotherapy often makes patients ill, anemic, and unable to combat infections.

The successes of prevention, surgery, radiation, and chemotherapy are often hidden by facts like those in Figure 3-3. They show that cancer has killed more and more people every decade since 1930. From these data, it would appear that the prevention and treatment of cancer has been ineffective. Let's analyze the situation, though. Figure 3-3 combines deaths from every kind of cancer. This is the sort of information you usually see. From it, you might conclude that all cancers are rising. But we could have declines in some offset by big rises in others. Figure 3-4 shows our suspicion is correct. The main cause of the overall rise in cancer deaths was the enormous rise in deaths from lung cancer. They have quadrupled since 1950. In contrast, deaths from colon cancer have fallen 27 percent, uterine cancer 73 percent, and stomach cancer 74 percent. Other cancers such as breast, prostate, ovarian, pancreatic, and leukemia rose slightly. If we omit lung

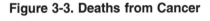

Figure 3-3. Deaths from Cancer

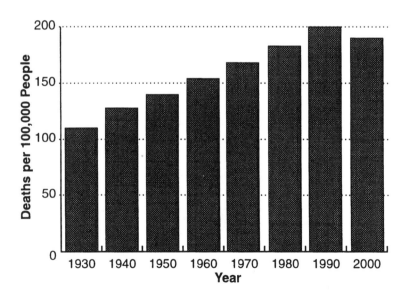

Figure 3-4. Deaths from Major Cancers

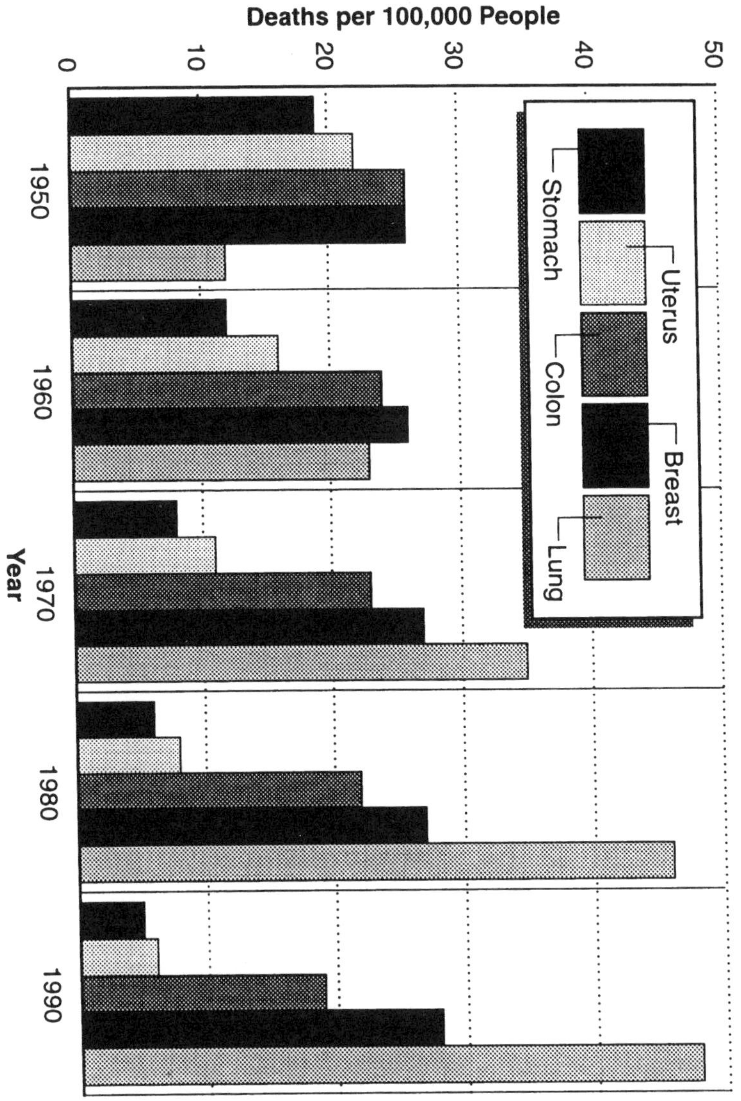

Deaths per 100,000 People

cancer, total cancer deaths have climbed only slightly since 1950.

Imagine how Figure 3-4 would look if no one smoked, eliminating almost all the lung cancer that now rears up highest among the bars. It would also prevent much of the stomach cancer and a fourth of the colon cancer. In addition, aspirin can prevent nearly half the remaining colon cancer, while a low-fat diet may prevent some breast and prostate cancer. It would certainly be a different picture.

Now, let's look in Figure 3-5 at the other powerful means to prevent deaths from cancer. You see the profound effect early detection has on the percentage of cases of the most common forms of cancer cured. For example, early detection results in the cure of 92 percent of colon cancer, but only 7 percent if it has spread. Even better, early detection leads to cures of 97 percent of breast cancer, 99 percent of prostate cancer, and 91 percent of ovar-

Figure 3-5. Cures from Early Detection

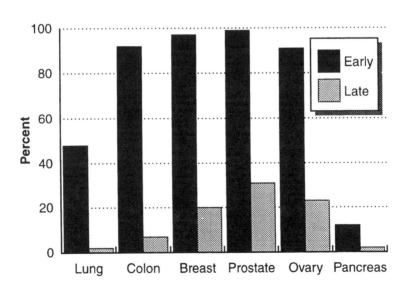

ian cancer. It also allows cures of more than 90 percent of melanoma, cervical, uterine, bladder, and testicular cancers. This doesn't mean all cancers can be treated so successfully. Figure 3-5 shows early detection cures only 48 percent of lung cancer and 10 percent of pancreatic cancer. Yet these cancers show little better than a 2 percent cure rate after they have spread. Even worse, glioblastoma, which comprises almost a third of brain cancers, is entirely fatal. Survival is estimated at less than a year after diagnosis. Thus, we have work to do.

Still, the outlook is bright. Between 1990 and 1995 deaths from lung cancer stopped rising and actually fell slightly. At the same time, the continued decline in deaths from other cancers caused a 3 percent drop in the total number of cancer related deaths for the first time in 60 years. According to these figures we can project a decreased number of deaths from cancer in the year 2000. If everyone used all of these preventive methods, including a thorough medical exam annually to improve early detection, we could wipe out 70 percent of cancer deaths. Prevention will improve as we discover more factors that cause cancer. In addition, research is uncovering new treatments that are likely to cure many cancers that have evaded prevention.

Experimental Advances In Treatment

We are now heading toward cures for cancer, even in advanced stages and without major side effects. Research in hundreds of laboratories is using our rising knowledge of molecular biology and immunology to devise ways to overcome cancer. Here are a few examples from different laboratories.

1. Researchers at the German Cancer Research Center have produced antibodies against lymphoma, a cancer of the lymph nodes or spleen. In the laboratory, the antibodies destroyed cancer cells. Injected into mice carrying hu-

man lymphoma, the antibodies destroyed the cancer. This may revolutionize treatment and act against many other cancers.

2. Researchers at Johns Hopkins Medical School have found that one cause of cancer is damage to tumor suppressor genes. In the laboratory, they inserted healthy tumor suppressor genes into colon cancer cells. The cells stopped growing. Insertion of the genes into bone cancer cells likewise stopped their growth. If we can insert tumor suppressor genes into cancer cells of patients, we may even stop widespread cancers.

3. Researchers at Temple University Medical School have made a DNA fragment that mirrors part of a growth gene that causes leukemia. In the laboratory, treatment of a mixture of leukemia and normal cells with the DNA fragment killed the leukemia cells but didn't harm normal cells.

4. Researchers at Harvard Medical School have devised a treatment for glioblastomas, fatal brain tumors. Since cancer cells in the brain divide, but normal cells don't, they made an altered form of a herpes virus that only attacks dividing cells. The virus killed glioblastoma cells in the laboratory. Injected into human glioblastomas in mice, the virus slowed the growth of the cancer and increased the survival rate of the mice.

5. Researchers at INSERM in Paris used the knowledge that glioblastoma cells make a lot of IGF-1 (Insulin-like Growth Factor 1), a protein which stimulates cell growth. By genetic engineering, they made cells that produce a DNA that mirrors the DNA for IGF-1 and ties up the gene. Injected into rats with glioblastomas in their brains, the cells caused the cancers to disappear within three weeks. The animals remained tumor-free during thirteen months of monitoring.

6. Researchers at Johns Hopkins Medical School have taken cells from kidney tumors in mice and have put genes

for interleukin-4, an immune substance, into them. When researchers injected the altered cells back into the mice, the animals developed an immunity to the cancer cells. The kidney tumors were destroyed.

7. Researchers at Scripps Research Institute have synthesized a new class of anticancer drugs more powerful than current ones. Unlike chemotherapy drugs, they kill cancer cells without harming normal cells. In laboratory tests, one was effective against pancreatic cancer, myeloma, and leukemia, cancers whose victims have poor survival rates.

8. Researchers at the Bristol-Myers Squibb Pharmaceutical Research Institute have made an antibody with affinity for many kinds of cancers. They attached a cell toxin, doxorubicin, to the antibody and injected it into mice afflicted with human lung, breast, or colon cancer. It cured all the cancers, even 70 percent of the lung cancer that had spread.

9. A dramatic advance in cancer cure came from the isolation of tumor suppressor genes whose damage cause many kinds of cancer. Researchers at the University of Texas M.D. Anderson Cancer Center inserted tumor suppressor genes into harmless viruses which then carried the genes inside cancer cells. When they injected the altered viruses directly into lung cancers in patients the cancers shrunk and disappeared. This technique should work with any solid tumor.

The potential of these treatments is impressive. They may take another ten years to get to physicians, however. Once there, they are likely to wipe out most cancers within a decade. In *Rx 2000* Dr. Fisher, with advice from dozens of researchers, predicts lung cancer deaths will fall 45 percent by the year 2002 and will be almost gone by 2025. Breast and colon cancer deaths will be rare by 2014. Prostate cancer deaths will fall 80 percent by 2012. All cancers will drop 75 percent by 2010 and will virtually be eliminated by 2030.

Rise in Life Expectancy from Progress Against Cancer

The prevention of cardiovascular disease can raise your life expectancy to age 87. The prevention of cancer does more to raise life expectancy further toward 100. Not smoking prevents 44 percent of deaths from cancer. When added to the prevention of deaths from cardiovascular disease, it raises life expectancy further.

■ Life expectancy of nonsmokers at age 35 = 91.

■ Life expectancy of nonsmokers at age 65 = 95.

■ Exercise prevents another 5 percent, aspirin 7 percent, and a low-fat diet 7 percent. Combined with early detection by medical exams, they prevent at least 70 percent of cancer.

■ Life expectancy of health-conscious 35-year-olds = 93.

■ Life expectancy of health-conscious 65-year-olds = 97.

Thirty-five-year-olds who use all the means to prevent and treat cardiovascular disease and cancer can expect to live almost 100 years. This puts them well into the era when we not only will have conquered most diseases but also will control aging.

The Road Ahead

Just like cardiovascular disease, cancer wouldn't be such a big barrier to longer life if everyone took these simple precautions to prevent it. Don't smoke. Avoid secondhand smoke. Have a medical exam annually. Use sunscreen. Eat a low-fat diet high in yellow and green vegetables. Take an aspirin tablet daily.

The problem again is that too many people kill themselves by failing to prevent cancer. They smoke, eat gobs of fat and deep-fried foods, never use sunscreen, and never go near a physician. Much of our death rate is due to neglect. If everyone acted to prevent cancer (especially by not smoking), it would not be nearly as big of a killer. Still, we can't prevent all cancers by these measures. There must be other agents that cause the cancers we can't prevent. There may be substances of which we are unaware in food, water, the atmosphere, medicines, beverages, or elsewhere in the environment that cause certain cancers. Some people are genetically prone to certain cancers. Whatever the case, one of our most important actions in the immediate future is to uncover the factors causing cancers we can't prevent today.

A vital search in the coming years will be for substances that prevent cancers. Vitamins E and C, beta-carotene, and selenium prevent the development of cancers in laboratory animals and are implicated in the prevention of human cancer. We must learn whether they prevent additional cancer in nonsmokers, and search for anticancer substances that are more effective treatments or prevention agents. We will develop more tests that detect various cancers early, eventually providing home diagnostic kits for cancer.

Since 1990, there has been an avalanche of laboratory success concerning new treatments for cancer. Many of these discoveries are now undergoing clinical tests on cancer patients. Some should be effective. In addition, continued research using specific antibodies, altered viruses, anticancer drugs, and gene therapy should give us powerful cures for cancer at any stage. It is likely that a whole array of new treatments, including specific antibodies against each kind of cancer and efficient drugs, will come into use between now and the year 2010. That should be the beginning of the end of cancer as a major disease. Progress in prevention and cure should continue until cancer is no longer a killer. In *Rx 2000* Dr. Fisher predicts an end to cardiovascular disease and cancer by the year 2030.

If we virtually eliminate cardiovascular disease and cancer by 2030, how much can we extend life? One group of researchers calculates it will raise life expectancy to age 99 and the maximum life span to 130. Using different assumptions, others estimate it will boost life expectancy at birth to 90. From standard life tables for the United States you can calculate it will raise life expectancy at birth to 98. Health-conscious 35-year-olds can expect to live to 104, 65-year-olds to 107, and 85-year-olds to 113.

It's difficult to predict when we will have the ability to conquer all cardiovascular disease and cancer. It could proceed steadily over several decades, or it could startle us with its rapidity. For example, recall the dramatic elimination of polio once a preventive vaccine was available. In five years, it was 90 percent gone. It has been expelled from the Western Hemisphere, and health workers are now moving to wipe it, like smallpox, from the face of the earth. Whether the control of cardiovascular disease and cancer is equally swift or proceeds steadily, by the year 2030 both will likely be under control or gone.

A 35-year-old's life expectancy of 93 is a second step in extending life. We can do more, however. We will see next how the prevention of other major diseases can extend your life to 100 or beyond.

4

Extending Life Beyond 100

We haven't found any biologic reason not to live to 110.
— Dr. Robert Butler, Former Director
National Institute on Aging

By preventing cardiovascular disease and cancer, you can raise your life expectancy to between 93 and 97 years. Ahead on the road to longer life, though, are barriers blocking your way to 100 and beyond. None is as massive as the two you have already overcome because none kills as many people as cardiovascular disease or cancer. But together, the eight strung out ahead of you cause 24 percent of all deaths—just as many as cancer causes. Before you lies the barrier of stroke, followed by chronic lung disease, accidents, pneumonia, diabetes, AIDS, suicide, and liver disease. As we reduce cardiovascular disease and cancer, people will live longer but will later fall victim to these or other diseases. Thus, stopping every disease is increasingly important. Biomedical researchers are advancing against almost all of them, even diseases that affect relatively few people. The total effect will be to extend life as far as we can before we find a way to control aging.

Stroke

Your third step to living longer is to prevent stroke. Most strokes occur when atherosclerosis narrows an artery and a clot blocks the flow of blood to the brain. The remainder occur when an artery bursts in the brain, often due to high blood pressure. Roughly a third of strokes are fatal, a third cause permanent injury, and a third have no lasting effect. If a stroke does not kill, it may paralyze one side of the body, making movement, swallowing, speech, and thought difficult. Strokes cause only 7 percent of deaths in the United States, but they are the top cause of serious disabilities.

There are three kinds of strokes. *Cerebral thrombosis* is a block in blood flow caused by a clot in the brain. *Cerebral embolism* is a block by a clot swept into the brain from elsewhere. *Cerebral hemorrhage* is the rupture of a blood vessel in the brain. Atherosclerosis is a cause of cerebral thrombosis and cerebral embolism. Hypertension is a cause of cerebral hemorrhage. Smoking, a previous heart attack, atrial fibrillation (a type of irregular heartbeat), a damaged heart valve, diabetes, and heavy drinking all raise the risk of stroke. Preventing stroke is much like preventing cardiovascular disease. Smokers have five times the risk of stroke of nonsmokers. But if smokers quit smoking, their risk decreases to nearly that of nonsmokers. Since atherosclerosis is the root cause of two-thirds of strokes, all the ways to prevent atherosclerosis also help prevent stroke. Strokes that arise from blood clots can be reduced by taking a 2.5-grain aspirin tablet daily. This will result in a 50-80 percent lower risk of these strokes. To reduce the risk of the one-third of strokes caused by hemorrhages in the brain, you must first curb hypertension by preventing atherosclerosis and obesity, avoiding stress, keeping salt low, avoiding lead, or by using an antihypertensive drug. Dietary potassium found in fruits and vegetables, especially bananas, reduces strokes. The potassium in one banana per day lowers your risk 40 percent. Heavy drinkers (10 ounces of alcohol per week) have four times the risk of stroke of nondrinkers. Surprisingly, light drinkers (0.5-3 ounces of alcohol per week) have half the risk of nondrinkers. As with cardiovascular disease, young women have fewer strokes than men. After menopause, women's strokes equal those of men. Low doses of estrogen prevent three-fourths of them, however. Altogether, these measures prevent 80 percent of strokes. You already use most of them.

There are increasing reports that persons taking a combination of vitamin E, vitamin C, and beta-carotene suffer half the strokes of persons who do not.

We should try to prevent strokes because treatment has lagged behind prevention. The best chance is a trip to an emergency room if you have dizziness, visual problems, slurred speech, loss of speech, difficulty in swallowing, or headaches. The clot-buster drug TPA can treat the two-thirds of strokes caused by blood clots. It's tricky to use, though, because it causes fatal bleeding in the one-third of strokes caused by hemorrhages and because it must be used within three hours of a stroke. If doctors diagnose a stroke, do a CT scan to rule out a hemorrhage, and give TPA at once, they can stop the stroke. More dazzling is a new drug, citicoline, which protects victims from brain damage after a stroke. In many cases, patients show almost complete recovery. The drug can be given within twenty-four hours of a stroke and still be effective. "This is definitely the most exciting time ever in the history of strokes," said Karen Putney, vice president of the National Stroke Association. This drug may revolutionize stroke treatment. Together with prevention, if may effectively wipe out deaths and infirmity from strokes.

In addition to citicoline, a series of new drugs that may prevent or repair stroke damage (Aptiganel, ZD9379, GV150-526A, Fosphenytoin, BW619-C89, SNX-111, Clomethiazole, Lubeluzole, Tirilazad, Enlimomab, and bFGF) are in or near clinical trials. Even if only a few are effective, when combined with rapid TPA therapy they should nearly wipe out injury from stroke.

Figure 4-1 shows that strokes kill fewer people each decade. If the trend continues, it projects deaths to be 25 percent of the rate of the 1950s by the year 2010 and gone by 2030.

The prevention of 80 percent of strokes extends life expectancy further beyond the 93 years attained by the prevention of cardiovascular disease and cancer.

- Life expectancy of health-conscious 35-year-olds = 95.
- Life expectancy of health-conscious 65-year-olds = 98.

Overcoming the barrier of stroke will bring your life expectancy closer to 100. It is easy to see why we have witnessed an explosive growth in the number of persons living past 90. You can push your life expectancy still closer to 100, though.

Figure 4-1. Stroke and Diabetes

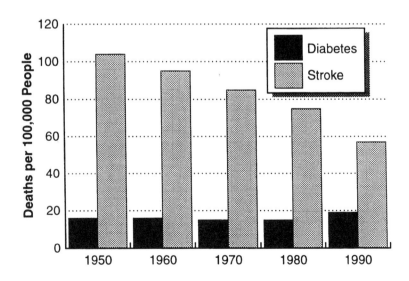

Chronic Lung Disease

Your fourth step to longer life is to jump over the hurdle of chronic lung disease. If you are a nonsmoker, it is easy. Let's look closely at this scourge that kills so many people. Chronic lung disease includes bronchitis, bronchial asthma, and emphysema. Chronic lung disease causes more than 4 percent of all deaths.

Bronchitis is an inflammation of the passages connecting the trachea to the lungs. Acute bronchitis is often a complication of a cold. With rest and treatment, it usually clears in a week. *Chronic bronchitis* is a persistent cough and breathlessness caused by inflammation. It leads to emphysema, pulmonary hypertension, and heart failure. *Bronchial asthma* is a difficulty in breathing, often of allergies to pollen, dust, dust mites, or cigarette smoke. It can appear early in life, then moderate or disappear in adult life. It causes only 7 percent of the deaths from chronic lung disease. *Emphysema* is the severe damage to the alveoli (air sacs) in the lungs. It leads to shortness of breath, respiratory or heart failure, and death. It is usually irreversible.

Smoking causes 85 percent of deaths from chronic lung disease. The other 15 percent are from air pollution. Many cases of asthma in children result from breathing secondhand smoke. Researchers have found that the exposure of children to tobacco smoke correlates with the occurrence and severity of asthma attacks. Children with the most exposure have twice the number of asthma attacks as those with least exposure to secondhand smoke.

Tobacco is again the source of a leading cause of death. It causes half the deaths from cardiovascular disease, nearly half from cancer, half from stroke, and now 85 percent from chronic lung disease. These are our first, second, third, and fourth leading causes of death. In view of the massive evidence that smoking is our biggest killer, it's astonishing that anyone smokes. Yet some smokers say they prefer to smoke, while some say they want to quit but can't. Tobacco may be addictive, and smokers drug addicts, not so different from cocaine or heroin addicts. In addition to the personal suffering caused by smoking, it also is the major reason for the high cost of health care.

Fortunately, growing numbers of people do not smoke. In 1950, 44 percent of United States adults smoked. By 1995, only 23 percent smoked. Figure 4-2 shows the progress. Tobacco has a bleak future. Bans on smoking are

Figure 4-2. Decline in Smoking

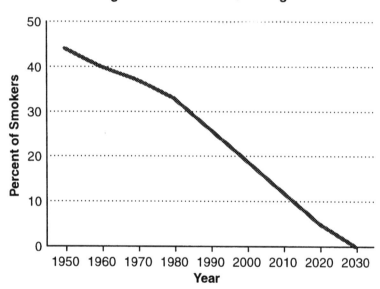

spreading. Taxes are rising. Smoking is becoming socially unacceptable. The number of smokers has dropped steadily. There may be only 19 percent of the population who smoke by the year 2000 and 12 percent by 2010. Smoking may be gone by 2030. It is the best thing that could happen to the nation's health. Nonsmokers can easily extend their life expectancy closer to 100 by preventing chronic lung disease.

■ Life expectancy of health-conscious 35-year-olds = 96.

■ Life expectancy of health-conscious 65-year-olds = 100.

Accidents

Your fifth step to longer life is to prevent accidents. They cause 4 percent of all deaths and are the leading cause of death for people under 35. Unlike diseases, accidents seem like a hodgepodge of happenings. Let's analyze them. Figure 4-3 shows the principal causes.

We see that a few actions can prevent most accidents. For example, accidents involving automobiles, trucks, and motorcycles cause the most deaths, but they result from surprisingly few causes.

■ Driving under the influence of alcohol causes 40 percent.

■ Excessive speed causes 27 percent.

■ Failure to yield right-of-way causes 11 percent.

■ All other lapses cause the remaining 22 percent.

Figure 4-3. Sources of Accidents

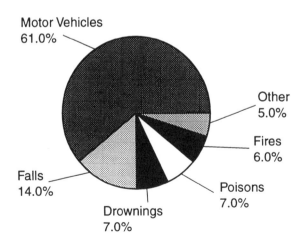

Hence, three factors cause more than three-fourths of the deaths from auto accidents. Avoid driving while intoxicated. To protect your life, governments have passed increasingly tough drunk driving laws, including big fines and the seizure of an intoxicated driver's license. To protect you from habitual drunks who drive after losing their licenses, there must be a mandatory confiscation of any vehicles they are caught driving. By barring drunk drivers from the road, we can lower accidental deaths 25 percent. Avoid excessive speed. To protect you from being killed by a speeder, fines for speeding must be high enough to stop them. Loss of license or automobile should be mandatory for repeat offenders. Reduction in speeding can reduce accidental deaths 14 percent. Defensive driving by you lowers it 8 percent more. Wear seat belts. There is strong evidence that seat belts save lives. Many vehicles have automatic seat belts. The United States National Highway Traffic Safety Administration has found that the use of seat belts causes an 11 percent drop in accidental deaths. Together, these few actions can eliminate more than half of all accidental deaths.

Falls cause 14 percent of accidental deaths and are often deadly for older adults. Twice as many persons past age 75 die from falls as from auto accidents. More than a third of falls break a hip, a wrist, or the spine. Death follows from infection of the fracture or from complications like pulmonary embolism, a blood clot in a lung. We can prevent falls with non-skid floors, especially in showers and bathtubs, along with the removal of throw rugs, protruding furniture, and icy steps and sidewalks. These measures can eliminate 8 percent of all accidental deaths.

Drownings cause 7 percent of accidental deaths. Most victims are males under 45. Many drownings are due to boating accidents. Also, many toddlers drown in swimming pools and bathtubs. A life jacket and the ability to swim will prevent most drownings. Constant attention to children in pools or tubs will prevent most other deaths from drowning.

Poisons cause 7 percent of accidental deaths, most of which either involve children who drink toxic chemicals or drug overdoses by addicts. There is no easy solution for addicts, but childproof containers can lower accidental deaths from poisoning by 4 percent.

We have the ability to wipe out 70 percent of deaths from accidents. Figure 4-4 shows the downward trend of deaths from accidents in the United States. From 1950 to 1980, they fell 25 percent, although deaths from vehicles stayed constant. Then, in the 1980s, accidental deaths fell

Figure 4-4. Downward Trend in Accidents

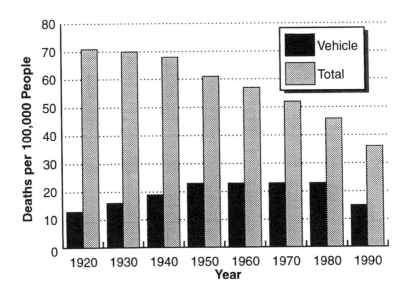

24 percent, including a 35 percent drop in deaths from motor vehicle accidents. This was probably due to seat belts and tougher laws against drunk driving.

By a few actions to prevent accidents, you can raise your life expectancy further.

- Life expectancy of health-conscious 35-year-olds = 97.
- Life expectancy of health-conscious 65-year-olds = 101.

Surmounting this barrier will take you into the vicinity of living 100 years.

Pneumonia And Influenza

Your sixth step toward long life is to prevent pneumonia and its frequent precursor, influenza. Pneumonia, an infection of the lungs, is our deadliest infectious disease. It causes 4 percent of all deaths. It is usually bacterial, but viruses and fungi can also cause it. The nasty thing about pneumonia is that its germs are everywhere. They enter your lungs when you inhale saliva or the mist expelled by people talking, sneezing, or coughing. The human immune system constantly fights off the infections. But in persons weakened by injury, surgery, diseases, or old age, pneumonia can develop fast. It is especially deadly in people over 65. Influenza is also dangerous. A virulent strain can appear anytime. In 1918, one such strain killed 20 million people, including half a million in the United States. It has not been as lethal recently, but that could change next year. Even in less lethal years, it kills many and is so debilitating that it often leads to pneumonia.

The sad thing about deaths from pneumonia and influenza is that we can prevent most of them. We have a growing set of weapons to prevent and treat both. A vaccine gives long-term protection from most pneumonia. Researchers have found it more than 60 percent effective, but few people become immunized. It makes no sense to avoid other diseases only to die of pneumonia. Annual immunization with a vaccine against the latest strains of influenza, especially in people over 65, is nearly 70 percent effective.

In turn, preventing influenza lowers the chance of getting pneumonia. A frequent cause of death from pneumonia is the failure to get medical help promptly. A bad cough, high temperature, painful breathing, or colored sputum should send you immediately to your physician. If diagnosed early, antibiotics and other treatments can overcome pneumonia. The same is true for influenza. Chills, fever, headache, muscle ache, and fatigue are classic symptoms of influenza (not of a cold) and should prompt you to get help from your physician. The antiviral drug amantadine, when given within twenty-four hours of the onset of illness, is highly effective at reducing the severity of influenza and lowering the risk of death. A newer drug, rimantidine, is even more effective.

Figure 1-1 shows how pneumonia deaths fell between 1920 and 1970. By 1980, they were only 14 percent of the number in 1920, but had risen again by 1990 in AIDS victims. Vaccines and prompt care can eliminate almost all deaths from pneumonia. Influenza vaccines and prompt treatment will do the same. Still, researchers are developing more effective vaccines against pneumonia and influenza. A new drug has given laboratory animals total protection against influenza. A vaccine based on viral DNA has given laboratory animals 90 percent protection from almost all strains of the influenza virus, raising the possibility of complete protection.

The big problem in resisting pneumonia, influenza, and other infectious diseases is the decline of our immune systems starting at age 20. Figure 4-5 shows the amazing drop.

By age 40, you have lost 25 percent of your immunity, by 65, 50 percent. By age 90, 80 percent of your immunity is gone. The astonishing thing is how steeply and how far it falls. This is our thin blue line against bacteria, viruses, fungi, protozoans, and all manner of savage creatures that continually try to kill us. By the time you reach 100, the

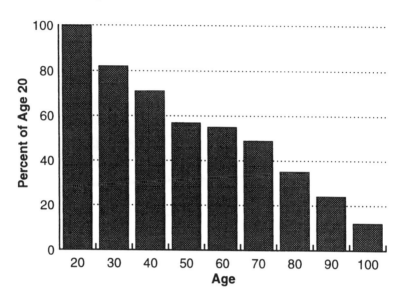

Figure 4-5. Decline in Immune Function

immune system striving desperately to protect you has only 10 percent of the strength it had at 20.

But researchers are progressing to restore lost immunity. They have found that regular injections of tiny doses of mercaptoethanol into old mice restores most of their lost immunity. Vitamin E also restores much of the immunity in aging rats. In a study of elderly people, 400 units of vitamin E per day gave markedly improved immunity. More surprising are the findings of two studies that a multivitamin tablet each day improves immune function greatly—in one study by a whopping 64 percent. Two studies found that 15-30 milligrams of zinc per day (many multivitamin tablets contain 15 milligrams) dramatically improve immune function. In another study of elderly persons, 20 milligrams of zinc produced a 50 percent increase in immune function. Vitamin E, multivitamins, and zinc appear so promising that you may want to supplement your diet with them. Vitamin

E already has been reported to prevent some cardiovascular disease and cancer, so it may be especially valuable for maintaining your health.

Thymosin is another substance that may keep immunity high. It is a hormonal protein produced by the thymus. As we age, the thymus deteriorates, thymosin production plummets, and immunity drops. Thymosin injections in laboratory animals and humans restore some of the lost immunity.

Prevention of these two diseases will take your life expectancy even higher.

- Life expectancy of health-conscious 35-year-olds = 98.

- Life expectancy of health-conscious 65-year-olds = 102.

Diabetes

Your seventh step to longer life is to prevent or control diabetes. In healthy people, the pancreas secretes *insulin*, a hormone that regulates the level of glucose in the blood. In diabetes, this process goes awry, causing 2 percent of all deaths.

Type I diabetes is insulin-dependent. *Type II diabetes* is not. According to the American Diabetes Association, 14 million Americans have diabetes. Many, who never go to a physician, aren't even aware of it. Of these, 13 million (93 percent) have type II diabetes. Only 7 percent have type I diabetes. Insulin-dependent diabetes occurs when your immune system destroys insulin-producing cells. It generally appears between ages 10 and 16. Without regular injections of insulin, the victim lapses into a coma and dies. Treatment requires a strict diet and insulin. Regulation of the insulin level is difficult. Even with insulin, difficulties like atherosclerosis, gangrene, and blindness can occur. There is no way to prevent or cure insulin-dependent diabetes. Type II diabetes has a gradual onset, usually after age 40. The body produces insulin but not enough to control the glucose level in the blood. This leads to the degeneration of blood vessels, blindness, kidney damage, and heart disease. The risk of type II diabetes is five times higher in obese persons. It is twice as likely in people over 55 or in people with hypertension. It is three times as likely if the parents are diabetic.

We can prevent many cases of Type II diabetes with a healthy lifestyle. Reduction of weight to the desirable level often wipes out type II diabetes without additional action. A balanced diet high in fruits and vegetables and the careful control of soluble sugars reduce the chance of a dangerous rise in blood glucose. Using up 1,000-1,500 calories per day through exercise lowers the risk of type II diabetes by 21 percent. Using up 2,000-2,500 calories reduces the risk 32 percent, while using up 3,500 calories almost cuts it in half. Preventing hypertension cuts in half the risk of developing type II diabetes. If other means of prevention aren't effective, oral drugs (tolbutamide, acetohexamide, chlorpropamide) usually will bring insulin back to a normal level.

Diet, exercise, and drugs can control almost all cases of type II diabetes. The real problem is the 7 percent of diabetes that is insulin-dependent. Scientists at Massachusetts General Hospital have masked human insulin-making cells with antibody fragments against the rejection mechanism in mice. When put into mice, the cells survived for the 200-day period of the experiment and produced human insulin during that time. If this procedure works in humans, it could eliminate daily insulin injections and return insulin production to normal. Researchers at the Washington University School of Medicine have enclosed rat insulin-making cells in hollow fibers of acrylic. When they put the fibers in diabetic mice, the plastic protected the insulin-making cells from the body's rejection mechanism. The cells produced a normal level of insulin over a 60-day period. The method is undergoing tests in humans.

Figure 4-1 shows the trend in deaths from diabetes between 1920 and 1990. Despite ways to eliminate most of the 93 percent of type II diabetes, deaths have risen in the United States. A major reason is the failure of people to have medical exams that diagnose diabetes before irreversible harm occurs. You can easily act to prevent type II diabetes with a yearly medical exam.

The prevention of type II diabetes alone can eliminate 90 percent of all deaths from diabetes, with a resulting increase in life expectancy.

■ Life expectancy of health-conscious 35-year-olds = 99.

■ Life expectancy of health-conscious 65-year-olds = 102.

Step by step, simple acts of prevention will take you past the barriers to longer life. Slowly but steadily, you will extend your life expectancy to 100.

AIDS

Your eighth step to living longer is to prevent AIDS, or acquired immune deficiency syndrome. It causes 1 percent of all deaths in the United States and infects more than a million people. It results from the infection of cells of the immune system by a human immunodeficiency virus (HIV). The AIDS virus does not kill directly. Instead, the victims, their immune system weakened by the virus, fall victim to pneumonia, tuberculosis, or other infectious diseases. Transmission of AIDS occurs most frequently through sexual intercourse and needle sharing by drug users, less often by the transfusion of AIDS-infected blood or by the accidental infection of health workers. AIDS spreads rapidly among people who have more than one sexual partner.

The frustrating thing about AIDS is that it is almost 100 percent preventable. Precaution in sexual intercourse and the rejection of needle sharing can eliminate 99 percent. Positive detection of contaminated blood can raise prevention to 100 percent. The problem is that too many people take no action to prevent AIDS.

As of 1996, there is no cure for AIDS. Drugs such as AZT slow the course of the disease but don't stop it. Research will develop a cure. It also may discover a preventive vaccine. If everyone tried, however, we could prevent almost all cases of AIDS today.

If you have avoided AIDS till now, you should be able to avoid it permanently, since we now know how to prevent it. This has a small effect on life expectancy.

- Life expectancy of health-conscious 35-year-olds = 99.
- Life expectancy of health-conscious 65-year-olds = 103.

Suicide

Your ninth step to longer life is to prevent suicide. Since you are reading a book on living longer, there is little chance that suicide is a threat to you. Suicide arises from complex psychological, social, and biological origins and causes 1 percent of all deaths. The highest rate is among older adults, but suicide has recently tripled among teenagers. Suicide notes tell us that suicide is often perceived by the victim as a way to escape an agonizing state of affairs or to wreak revenge on someone blamed for the victim's suffering. The victim feels life is so painful that only death can provide relief. Depression is also a factor in most suicides. Some people may be more genetically inclined to depression than others. Depression often results from chronic pain or a staggering problem like isolation, the death of a loved one, a broken home, illness, old age, unemployment, financial trouble, drug addiction, or psychiatric illness.

The first step in preventing suicide is to recognize severe depression. A relative, friend, or even the victim may suspect it. Recognition should lead one to seek help. Vigorous action against depression has become an important means to prevent suicide. The most effective preventive treatment has been the drug fluoxetine (Prozac), which also has the fewest side effects. It prevents depression in an astounding 70 percent of cases and is estimated to prevent many suicides. New drugs are appearing that may be even more effective. Antidepressant drugs are important, but psychiatric treatment is essential. A combination of psychiatric treatment and drugs can prevent most suicides. Limit access to guns by depressed persons. Surprisingly, researchers have found a five times greater risk of suicide in people who live in homes with firearms.

Preventing suicide should be a freebie for you. Since suicide causes only 1 percent of all deaths, its prevention has a minimal effect on life expectancy. This still extends life expectancy another year.

- Life expectancy of health-conscious 35-year-olds = 100.
- Life expectancy of health-conscious 65-year-olds = 103.

Chronic Liver Disease

The tenth step to living longer is to prevent chronic liver disease. It causes 1 percent of all deaths. Most are due to cirrhosis and hepatitis. A few deaths result from poisoning by excess acetaminophen, cancer, autoimmune attack, hemochromatosis, or Wilson's disease. *Cirrhosis* results from chronic damage to liver cells by alcohol and other toxic agents and by the diseases of the liver listed above. Alcohol is a powerful poison in the liver, so heavy drinking is the biggest source of cirrhosis. *Hepatitis* is an inflammation of the liver from hepatitis viruses or other causes. Chronic hepatitis usually leads to cirrhosis.

You can prevent 80 percent of liver disease by avoiding heavy drinking. You can further prevent it by avoiding infection by viral hepatitis B from sexual activity, needles, and ear piercing and by avoiding excess acetaminophen. Immunization against the hepatitis B virus is effective.

■ The damage of cirrhosis is irreversible. If the cirrhosis is caused by alcohol abuse, cessation of drinking stops further degradation of the liver. Other causes of cirrhosis are often treatable, but the major way to wipe out most deaths from liver disease is to avoid heavy drinking. As long as you don't drink heavily, you stand a good chance of avoiding liver disease. This adds another year to your life expectancy.

■ Life expectancy of health-conscious 35-year-olds = 101.

■ Life expectancy of health-conscious 65-year-olds = 104.

Rise in Life Expectancy from the Prevention of Diseases and Accidents

Step by step, your actions to prevent diseases and accidents can raise your life expectancy to between 101 and 104 years. Though most people don't use all of these preventive measures, a growing number use many. It is easy to understand why people over 85 and over 100 are the fastest-growing age groups today. If you were 35 in 1990 and use all preventive measures against the ten barriers to longer life, you could expect to live until the year 2056. By then, we will be capable of controlling aging. You could live right past 2100. Even if you were 65 in 1990, you could expect to live until 2029. Initial control of aging may permit you also to live past the year 2100.

The Road Ahead

The actions we take to prevent the leading causes of death and extend healthy life are amazingly similar. Not smoking, that great preventer of cardiovascular disease and cancer, prevents half of stroke and 85 percent of chronic lung disease. Exercise, a low-fat diet, and the control of obesity and hypertension help prevent stroke and most diabetes. A sensible lifestyle, including immunization and medical exams, goes far toward extending healthy life past 100.

It does not stop there. Research on the many diseases we face is forging ahead. The continuation of rapid advances since 1980 projects a growing ability to prevent or cure all the top killers. Stroke should drop with cardiovascular disease. Chronic lung disease should succumb to a drop in smoking. Accidents should fall due to engineering, better laws, and education. Pneumonia should yield to better vaccines and drugs. Diabetes should fade with healthy lifestyles and drugs for type II, plus genetic therapy or drugs for type I. AIDS should abate when research produces vaccines. Suicide should fall as a result of better health care. The top killers should decline until we have the ability to nearly eliminate them by the year 2030.

If conquering the ten leading killers raises life expectancy to between 101 and 104 years, what happens as we eliminate additional diseases? The next five killers—numbers eleven through fifteen—are homicide, kidney disease, miscellaneous infectious diseases, septicemia (massive bacterial infection), and the diseases of infancy. They cause another 5 percent of all deaths. Research is progressing against them all. As we reduce them, health-conscious 35-year-olds can expect to live to age 102, and 65-year-olds to 105. But a life expectancy of 102 is not the limit. Research is attacking the 100 diseases that cause 99 percent of deaths and will push your life expectancy toward age 120. It's a bright outlook.

5

Your Inner Longevity Factor

*A strong will to live, along with the other positive
emotions—faith, love, purpose, determination, humor—
are biochemical realities that can affect
the environment of medical care.*
—Norman Cousins, *Head First*

Although the ability of biomedical research to extend your
life is astounding, its success depends ultimately on you.
It takes willpower to stop smoking, exercise daily, or keep
your weight in the desirable range. If you hate needles, it
takes teeth-gritting resolve to immunize yourself against
pneumonia and influenza, even though the needles are now
so thin you can hardly feel them. If you have the determination, preventive measures can boost your life expectancy past
100. Research is charging forward to find ways to prevent
even more diseases. Together with the many advantages bio-
medicine gives you are the added factors of willpower, love
of life, will to live, and inner spirit. They are immensely
important for a long, healthy life. Whether you call your
impetus resolve, determination, willpower, or spirit, it is *yours*
to use because it is deeply rooted inside your mind.

The Mind-Body Connection

We sometimes forget that our mind not only receives input from our senses, but also connects, by means of an intricate network of nerves, to every organ and tissue throughout the body. A liver, heart, kidney, or stomach does not operate independently. These and all other organs are controlled by your brain. As a result, the brain can produce myriad effects. For example, Susan's heart skipped a beat at the sight of Wolfgang's rippling muscles. Her heart really did skip a beat—probably several. Susan's visual input to her brain of those enticing muscles caused it to respond by, among other actions, sending a signal to her heart that disturbed its rhythm.

Input from your senses to your brain can trigger far more violent reactions than a skipped heartbeat. How do you react to buckets of blood all over the road at the scene of an auto accident? Do you turn cold and vomit? Would you do the same if you were trapped inside a vat of rotting flesh? In these cases, signals from sensory cells in your eyes or nose cause your brain to send a command to your stomach. Motion sickness is a similar reaction. Conflicting signals sent to your brain from your eyes and inner ear provoke a reaction that makes some people so ill that it can be life threatening. In contrast, soft music can calm us, lowering pulse and blood pressure as the ear signals the brain, which orders the rest of the body to relax.

Power of the Mind To Cause Bodily Harm

Some effects produced by your brain are far more serious than motion sickness. There is startling evidence that negative emotional states trigger disabling effects on your immune system, heart function, and even on the development of cancer. Chief among these is stress.

Stress is any stimulus causing mental or emotional disruption capable of affecting physical health. It usually produces an increased heart rate, a rise in blood pressure, muscular tension, irritability, and depression. Stress occurs in three stages. The first is alarm, when your body detects stress and prepares for action, basically to fight or escape. You release hormones to increase heartbeat and respiration. You boost blood sugar for quick energy. You perspire. (Remember the cold sweat of horror novels?) Your pupils dilate. Your digestion slows. Alarm can make you nauseated. These are savage effects on your body, but they have evolved as a way to mobilize your resources to save your life when you round a corner and come face-to-face with a saber-toothed tiger. The second stage is resistance, when your body repairs damage caused by alarm. If stress continues, your body remains tense and can't repair the damage. The third stage, exhaustion, results from continued stress. A stress-related disorder can arise. Prolonged stress depletes the body's energy and affects bodily functions so severely that it can cause even death.

Our intense reaction to stress may have evolved from the need of early humans to be constantly on guard for threats from wild animals, natural hazards, and other people. To cope with these, the body has evolved quick reactions—fight or flight. The heart races, blood pressure jumps, hormones pour into the bloodstream to command the body's organs to meet the threat. Action against the threat—running away or fighting—causes the body's systems to return to normal. Yet problems occur when the body is prepared to cope with trouble but can't. Being caught in a traffic jam on the way to the airport for a vital trip, a missed flight connection costing you something important, a holdup, or even morning traffic can cause your body to activate a flight-or-fight response. But when you can take no action, the systems remain in a high state of readiness. Constant repetition of extended high states of readiness interferes with the proper operation of vital systems in your body, and produces physical illness.

Cardiovascular Disease

The most common effect of mental stress is to increase hypertension. Less well known are findings by Dr. Alan Rozanski and his colleagues at the UCLA School of Medicine that stress causes substantial and usually imperceptible myocardial ischemia, insufficient blood flow to the heart. Even less well known is that stress is a factor in blood cholesterol level. Although cholesterol level is usually associated only with diet, many researchers have shown that stress produces abnormally high cholesterol levels in the blood. This, of course, is a factor in accelerating atherosclerosis, the root cause of most cardiovascular disease. Hence, your mind can cause severe damage to your cardiovascular system. Even more ominous is the conclusion of researchers that emotional stress triggers 40 percent of all cases of cardiac arrest. A dramatic instance of this occurred during the Los Angeles earthquake of 1994. Physicians found five times as many people died from cardiac arrest on the day of the earthquake as ordinarily do. Two-thirds of those died within an hour of the quake.

Stress can affect the heart in several ways. It can influence the heart's rhythm. It can break loose a lump of fatty buildup in an artery, causing a heart attack. It can also cause a spasm in an artery to squeeze off the blood supply to the heart.

Immune Function

The immune system reacts strongly to stress. For example, researchers have found that several kinds of stress all cause a striking reduction in the components of the immune system and an increase in the presence of latent viruses. Likewise, mental depression is associated with the reduced activity of the immune system's natural killer cells, and it also accelerates the spread of tumors in breast cancer patients.

Cancer

Cancer results from damage to DNA. Most DNA damage is repaired quickly by the body's DNA repair system. In highly depressed patients, DNA repair is much worse than in nondepressed patients. In fact, DNA repair and resistance to cancer correlates with the extent of depression. The worse the depression, the poorer the repair.

Other Diseases

Headaches, facial pain, back pain, and premenstrual stress are frequent stress-generated disorders. Stress also can cause skin disorders, including itching, rashes, or pimples.

More serious are gastrointestinal problems such as ulcers. Ulcers are caused by an infection of the stomach by a bacterium, *Helicobacter pylori*. Stress produces excess gastric juice and changes in the stomach lining that aid the invasion by Helicobacter pylori. The resulting ulcers cause the nausea and pain characteristic of the disease. Other stress-related gastrointestinal diseases involve inflammation of the colon and bowels, such as enteritis or the more serious ulcerative colitis. Anorexia nervosa, a refusal to eat even to the point of death (usually by teenage girls) is also the result of stress. Bulimia nervosa is a related malady in which stress from abnormal concern over weight and figure by teenage girls causes repeated episodes of bingeing on food and then vomiting.

Respiratory disorders are frequently affected by stress. The most common is asthma, in which emotional upsets bring on attacks characterized by wheezing, panting, and feeling suffocated.

Thus, one's state of mind has a vast ability to produce harmful, even fatal, effects on the body's physiology. For long life, it is essential to avoid depression and continued stress. This takes a big effort in today's society. The effect of one's mental state on illness is so well established that a new branch of medicine, behavioral medicine, has appeared. Behavioral medicine concerns the effects of behavior on health and illness. It deals with the occurrence, prevention, and control of physical disorders caused or aggravated by social interactions, thought, and emotions. Researchers in behavioral medicine study how stress produces disease, how placebos work, how pain can be regulated, and how patients can prevent mentally-caused illnesses.

Power of the Mind to Contribute to Well-Being

Your mind has much power to cause physical harm, but it also has astounding power to help prevent and fight diseases. Studying the *placebo effect* is one of the ways researchers first observed the power of the mind in treating diseases. In a great number of studies, patients given a sugar pill but told it is a powerful drug for their illness showed measurable improvement. In a striking case, patients were told that they could expect hair loss from chemotherapy. A third of the patients receiving a placebo lost their hair. Placebos have never been demonstrated to cure a disease, but improvement is common. This is another indicator that the mind has a powerful effect on physiology.

The idea that the mind, through a determined and positive attitude, can influence the course of a disease received an enormous boost from the widely read experience of Norman Cousins, former editor of *Saturday Review*. In his book *Anatomy of an Illness*, he tells in stirring detail of the helpful effect a positive attitude and a close partnership with his physician had on his recovery from a serious illness. Since then, numerous studies have defined the role that a positive, determined outlook by both patient and physician has as an aid to standard therapy. A surprising finding has been the value of humor and laughter. Researchers have found that a large dose of humor often reduces the severity of a disease and may even help prevent some diseases. Just as stress, depression, or other negative factors are physically detrimental, positive factors have been shown to improve therapy and prevent disease. Researchers have found that the survival of women who have undergone breast cancer surgery is more common in those showing a "fighting spirit" than in those with a "hopeless" attitude. In another study, researchers have found that patients with a positive attitude have better immune functions and slower growth of the deadly tumors of malignant melanoma compared to patients with a passive outlook. These findings of the benefit of a positive outlook have been confirmed by many researchers on many kinds of cancer. For example, a survey of 690 oncologists concerning more than 10,000 cancer patients has revealed that treatment is more effective, and recovery more likely, in patients with a strong will to live, hopefulness, coping ability, and a cooperative relationship with their physicians.

But mental attitude is not a universal panacea. Researchers have found in advanced, high-risk cancer that the biology of the cancer determines the outcome no matter how positive the attitude. There is no evidence that one can simply cure any disease, no matter how advanced, with the mind alone. Mental factors appear to operate best either in the prevention of illnesses or in the cure of early to moderately advanced diseases.

We saw earlier that depression or stress lowers immune activity. An exciting finding is that a positive outlook not only prevents reduced immunity but also in many cases actually increases the production of immune cells. This means that a cheerful, positive attitude helps keep your immune system at its optimal state to ward off disease. Studies also show that a positive outlook can act as a buffer to protect you from lowered immunity during periods of stress. One of the most astonishing findings concerns the immune system in elderly people. You will recall from chapter 4 that our immunity declines throughout life. By the time people reach age 80 their immune system averages only 30 percent of what it was at age 20. In elderly persons with a positive attitude and "emotional hardiness" toward events in life, researchers have found immunity comparable to that of younger people. In addition to a positive outlook, physical exercise contributes to higher immune function. Researchers have also found depression suppresses immunity increasingly with advancing age. It may contribute significantly to the lower immunity we see during aging. These findings are extremely important because a progressively higher barrier to longer life as you get older is infectious disease, chiefly from a weaker immune system. Anything that helps keep immunity high will extend life.

It's All Up To You

Determination, spirit, and an optimistic outlook can help you avoid the harmful effects of depression and stress. More important, the same characteristics can contribute mightily to the prevention and cure of diseases. They can increase immune function, aid in overcoming cancer and other diseases, and promote healing. They even appear to slow some of the deterioration of aging. Although much research is underway, we have not uncovered the full potential of a positive mental attitude or how to unleash it for maximum effect in curing disease. Much is still not understood about the effects of the mind and spirit on the body. There is little doubt that good humor and a positive outlook are your best allies when medicine works to prevent or treat a disease. These qualities are in your hands. Above all, you need a relentless determination to live. Never forget William Henley's defiant words from *Invictus*: "I am the master of my fate. I am the captain of my soul."

6

How Far Can Medicine Go?

*The power of molecular medicine is now so great that
there is no disease it cannot face.*
—Bernadine Healy, M.D.
Former Director, U.S. National Institutes of Health

A 100-year life is not your limit. Each year, your ability to live even longer will climb as medicine conquers more diseases and surgery repairs hurts that were hopeless a few years ago. Within several decades, your life expectancy will shoot upward when biomedical scientists begin to control aging. But let's look first at how much you can extend life *only* by overcoming diseases. To do it, we must answer two questions:

**As your life expectancy rises past 100,
what diseases may you face?**

**How far can medicine go to wipe out
these diseases and all other diseases?**

We will look first at the diseases you may face. Then we will see where medicine is going to overcome these and all other diseases.

Barriers Beyond 100

What barriers to longer life will you face when you are past 100? One way to consider possibilities is to see what diseases are barriers for the "oldest of the old." After 85, deaths from cardiovascular disease and cancer drop. It isn't clear why, but they do. People over 85 are also less likely to be killed by auto accidents, chronic lung disease, diabetes, liver disease, AIDS, or homicide. In their places, other diseases become more important. More deaths at this age result from pneumonia, pulmonary embolism, septicemia, Alzheimer's disease, and from broken bones and surgery.

Several researchers have studied the causes of death of people over 85. Figure 6-1 shows that the barriers to longer life change markedly from those for younger persons.

Even combined, cardiovascular disease and stroke drop from causing half the deaths to causing less than a fourth.

Figure 6-1. Barriers Beyond Age 85

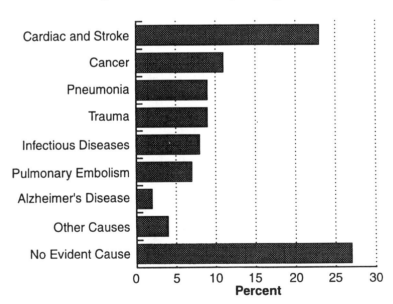

Cancer causes only a bit more than 10 percent. But deaths are three times higher from pneumonia and eight times higher from other infectious diseases, due to lower immunity. Trauma from surgery or broken bones causes fatal blood clots or infections. Pulmonary embolism (a blood clot blocking an artery to the lungs) is a threat. Alzheimer's disease causes 2 percent of deaths. Most deaths of people over 85 are due to no evident cause. Aging probably causes these. As you live past 85, you increasingly face the ultimate killer, aging. Aging causes cells to deteriorate to a point where they stop working. No one has ever survived this condition.

Aging limits how far medicine can extend life by curing diseases. Long life depends on the prevention or cure of diseases, but somewhere in the 100-130 year range we must control aging if we are to extend life further. But first, as cardiovascular disease, cancer, and stroke fade as threats to you past 100, let's look more closely at the five diseases that may be your major barriers to still longer life. We will also see how much the prevention or cure of these and other diseases will raise life expectancy beyond 100.

Pneumonia

Here is pneumonia again, a bigger threat to you past 85. But immunization against pneumonia and influenza can prevent many cases. Prompt treatment with antibiotics can cure more. Strengthening your immune system with a daily multivitamin tablet containing 400 units of vitamin E and 20 milligrams of zinc can help both the prevention and cure. Thus, pneumonia may not be so big a threat if you are prepared.

Other Infectious Diseases

Over age 85, a weak immune system that is a big factor in pneumonia extends to dozens of other infectious diseases. Diseases that you would have thrown off easily in youth suddenly threaten your life. Especially dangerous is septicemia, or blood poisoning, in which infective bacteria (in an abscess, urinary tract infection, intestinal infection, or other site) secrete poisons into the bloodstream. You can reduce this threat by consciously avoiding infection, keeping immunity high, and getting prompt treatment for any infection.

Trauma From Surgery Or Bone Fractures

Here is a third threat from bacterial infection—this time from the infection of a surgical wound or bone fracture. Again, the culprit is a weak immune system. Surgeons can minimize infection by treating you with antibiotics before surgery. You can reduce bone fractures by removing the causes of falls, by using drugs to lessen the loss of balance due to aging, and by retarding *osteoporosis*, a loss of protein from the bones that causes them to become brittle. In osteoporosis, protein loss begins around age 30. By age 80, women have lost 28 percent of bone tissue and men 14 percent. Bones break from falls that would have no effect on a younger person. But you can slow protein loss with dietary calcium from milk and other foods, plus moderate activity. Estrogen therapy after menopause slows osteoporosis in women and cuts fractures 50 percent. Sodium etidronate, a drug promoting bone formation, also reduces osteoporosis and halves bone fractures.

Pulmonary Embolism

A different threat to you past age 85 is a block in the pulmonary artery or its branches in the lungs by an *embolus*, often a blood clot. In the pulmonary artery, a clot can cause instant death. If not, physicians can destroy it with clot-busting drugs. The anticoagulants heparin or dicumarol can prevent additional clots.

In younger adults, clots arise from surgery or pregnancy. Getting out of bed and being active minimizes clots. In older adults, the clot often arises from deep vein thrombosis, when sitting still for long periods causes clots to form in the legs. Active elderly people have little pulmonary embolism. But immobility rises with strokes, congestive heart failure, and arthritis. Stroke victims need physical therapy to become as active as possible. Victims of congestive heart failure can use diuretics, vasodilators, and digitalis to combat fatigue and become active until a cure is possible. Arthritis victims can use drugs to suppress pain and oral doses of type II collagen, a protein, to improve most arthritis and possibly give total relief. In addition, researchers have found that vitamin C (1 gram per day) prevents deep vein thrombosis. Since aspirin also inhibits clot formation, a combination of activity, vitamin C, and aspirin can prevent most deaths from pulmonary embolism.

Alzheimer's Disease

Except for aging, your toughest barrier to longer life past 85 is Alzheimer's disease. This progressive degeneration of brain cells is invariably fatal. It afflicts 4 million people in the United States and causes 14,000 deaths per year. Alzheimer's disease has appeared as early as age 28, but it is mostly a disease of advanced age. Figure 6-2 shows its spectacular increase with age. It afflicts few 65-year-olds, but by the time they are 90, one-third of them are victims of Alzheimer's disease. Although it soars with advanced age, there is no evidence it is caused by the aging process. The cause lies elsewhere.

The characteristics of Alzheimer's vary, but it develops in three stages. In the *early stage*, victims are increasingly forgetful. They may try to overcome it by writing reminder lists or covering memory lapses. They feel anxious. In the *middle stage*, forgetfulness changes to severe memory loss, especially for recent events. Victims become disoriented and lose their way on familiar streets. The ability to do simple mathematics degrades. (This is an important symptom.) They can't concentrate. As the disease develops further, victims can't find the right words to speak. Anxiety

Figure 6-2. Age and Alzheimer's Disease

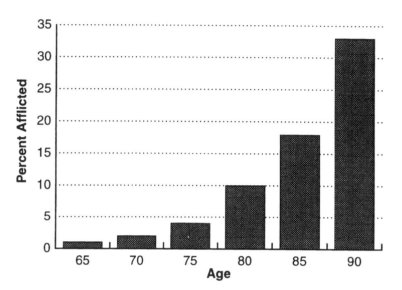

heightens as they realize something is wrong. They become depressed and subject to sudden swings in mood. In the *final stage*, victims become severely disoriented and confused, often unable to recognize family members. Some are demanding, others docile and helpless. They suffer delusions and hallucinations. They lose control of bodily functions and jerk involuntarily in the manner of newborns. Eventually they are bedridden, completely helpless, and die of pneumonia, infections, or other complications.

Being forgetful is not necessarily a sign that you are getting Alzheimer's. We sometimes are all forgetful. We forget how forgetful we are. Teenagers are conveniently forgetful. Scientists are hilariously forgetful. We just go on writing reminders.

Alzheimer's disease occurs in two forms: early onset (hereditary) and late onset. *Early-onset Alzheimer's* is uncommon. It is inherited through families due to a defective gene. A feature of early-onset Alzheimer's is its appearance by age 40, although victims are often younger. Almost all Alzheimer's cases in young persons are hereditary. Victims usually die within ten years of diagnosis. *Late-onset Alzheimer's* occurs far more often. Figure 6-2 shows it occurs mostly after age 70. The notable factor in late-onset Alzheimer's is age. Head injury, lack of education, and heart attack are risk factors, but age is the big thing. Late-onset Alzheimer's usually proceeds within a few years to death, although medical treatment may extend a victim's life ten years. There are few diagnostic tests for the disease, although poor linguistic ability early in life seems to be an uncanny predictor of later development.

A startling finding is that the drug ibuprofen, an ingredient in many headache remedies, may reduce the risk of developing Alzheimer's by as much as 60 percent. Aspirin and acetaminophen have no effect. Even one ibuprofen tablet per week is effective. A study of more than 2,000 elderly persons by researchers at Johns Hopkins University provides evidence that anti-inflammatory drugs somehow prevent the formation of protein plaques that accumulate in the brains of Alzheimer's victims. It agrees with a study at Duke University of fifty sets of twins. The study found that the twins who took an anti-inflammatory drug were ten times less likely to develop Alzheimer's. Thus, we have aspirin to prevent cardiovascular disease and colon cancer and ibuprofen to prevent Alzheimer's disease.

We should try to prevent Alzheimer's because we can't yet cure it. Tacrine (tetrahydroaminoacridine), the first drug to act against the disease, slows it almost 10 percent. This is a small reduction, but it's a first step and a harbinger of more effective drugs. It also buys time as researchers try to understand the disease enough to find out how to overcome it.

To conquer Alzheimer's, we must first understand it. We now know something of the events in the brain during the development of the disease. Victims' brains shrink, and there is a marked decline in substances that transmit nerve impulses. But the most visible change is the destruction of brain tissue, which fills with tangles of protein fibers that replace brain cells and plaques of insoluble protein among the dying brain cells. *Tangles* consist mainly of an abnormal form of a protein that is found in microtubules, the tubular girders that support the structure of brain cells. In Alzheimer's, many units of this abnormal protein combine to produce bizarre tangles. *Plaques* are masses of ß-amyloid, a small, abnormal protein. Thus, terrible things happen in the brains of victims of Alzheimer's disease. Something kills areas of their brain cells and causes normal proteins to become the plaques and tangles of abnormal proteins. As this occurs, victims steadily lose touch with everything.

A major advance against Alzheimer's disease is the discovery that at least some Alzheimer's—like cancer, cystic fibrosis, multiple sclerosis, and many other diseases—is caused by damage to one or more genes. This is important because identification of the genes will lead to the conquest of the disease.

Early-onset Alzheimer's results from damage to a single gene. The gene can be on chromosome 1, chromosome 14, or chromosome 21. The chromosome 1 and chromosome 14 genes are linked to a curious process in our bodies, *programmed cell death*. Your body can have unneeded cells. When it does, it signals the cells to kill themselves. A group of genes in each cell initiates and oversees the cell's death and disintegration. Thus, each of your cells contains a death mechanism that would make for a creepy science fiction story. The genes on chromosomes 1 and 14 causing Alzheimer's are essentially identical to genes that keep programmed cell death switched off. The defective form of these genes may no longer prevent cell death in the brain, causing Alzheimer's. The location of the other Alzheimer's-causing gene on chromosome 21 is noteworthy because the gene causing Down's syndrome is also on chromosome 21. Down's syndrome victims often get Alzheimer's disease by the time they reach 35. The gene normally is the pattern for *amyloid precursor protein* (APP). The cell cuts APP to form one or more smaller proteins. APP is cut to form the smaller protein nexin-2, a protein that stops the breakdown of other proteins and helps form ties between nerve endings in the brain. But if the APP gene is damaged, it produces a Frankenstein APP that is cut in the wrong places to form ß-amyloid, the protein forming plaques in the brains of Alzheimer's victims. Normally, when APP is cut to form nexin-2, the cut goes through the ß-amyloid portion and destroys it.

In the laboratory, ß-amyloid is a ravenous killer of nerve cells. It may do the same in the brain. This could be one of the results of the damaged gene on chromosome 21.

Late-onset Alzheimer's may also result from damage to genes, but we don't yet know. Which genes and how they relate to genes for early-onset Alzheimer's are important questions. Some people may carry genes that make them more susceptible to Alzheimer's. Whatever the case, the older one gets, the more likely genes are to be damaged. This might explain the increase in Alzheimer's disease with age.

Although Alzheimer's disease is the most intractable malady faced by 100-year-olds, progress against it has been rapid. A simple test to detect it has appeared. More drugs to slow its progress are being developed. Identification of the causative genes can lead to a cure by replacing the damaged genes with normal ones or by developing a drug that bypasses the damaged genes. For the growing numbers of health-conscious people who live past 100, Alzheimer's disease should fade as a threat.

How Far Can Medicine Go?

The biggest barriers to longer life for younger people—

cardiovascular disease, cancer, and stroke—become progressively smaller as you pass age 80 and head for 100. Even diseases that become larger barriers for you after age 85 pneumonia, other infectious diseases, trauma from injury or surgery, and pulmonary embolism, can be prevented or treated successfully with your efforts. Hence, the outlook for you past 100 is surprisingly bright.

But there are still barriers. The most visible is Alzheimer's disease. In addition, recall that 100 diseases cause 99.9 percent of deaths. We have looked at no more than 20 of the 100. The remaining 80 are responsible for only a fraction of the trouble caused by the top 20, but among them are potential problems for you as you live beyond 100.

Against these problems, however, is the power of an incredible juggernaut of biomedical research. It is producing a stream of tests and instruments to diagnose diseases and is using the power of computers to aid in diagnosis. It is developing ever better medications to combat a hundred diseases, including drugs to wipe out antibiotic-resistant bacteria. Researchers have identified genes responsible for cystic fibrosis, multiple sclerosis, muscular dystrophy, amyotrophic lateral sclerosis, and other diseases that have seemed incurable. Human trials are underway to replace flawed genes in a dozen hereditary diseases, and these will move quickly toward therapy for all hereditary diseases. Engineers are producing a growing number of mechanical body parts, but they likely will be superseded by human organs grown in culture. Biomedical firms already grow human skin for burn victims, and this is leading to the growth of livers to replace diseased ones. Hearts, kidneys, and other organs are not far behind. Each week, biomedical journals report advances toward the prevention or cure of diseases. Some are part of a step-by-step progress toward a success ten years in the future. Others are astounding conquests that were unthinkable a few years ago.

How far can medicine go? Like the 500-pound gorilla, it can go as far as it wants. All evidence is that medicine will overcome the leading causes of death in the next few decades, and conquer, during the twenty-first century, diseases that now cause 99 percent of all deaths. We face the awesome reality of an approaching time when medicine can prevent and cure almost all diseases.

Increased Life Expectancy from Overcoming Diseases

If health-conscious people avoid the leading killers, what happens to life expectancy as we control the remaining diseases? Within several decades, medicine should have the ability to prevent or cure 25 percent of all known diseases, including cancer, cardiovascular disease, stroke, diabetes, Alzheimer's disease, cystic fibrosis, multiple sclerosis, muscular dystrophy, and most microbial infections. Their conquest (not including the control of aging) will push life expectancy past 100.

- Health-conscious 35-year-olds can expect to live to 104.
- Health-conscious 65-year-olds can expect to live to 106.

If at the same time we begin to control aging, your life expectancy will rise far above 104 or 106.

Continued research will give medicine the power to prevent or cure 50 percent of all known diseases. Although we probably will have learned to slow aging by then, the conquest of more diseases will further contribute to the rise in life expectancy.

- Health-conscious 35-year-olds can expect to live to 107.
- Health-conscious 65-year-olds can expect to live to 109.

If you are health conscious, by the time you reach 100 you can expect to live on to 115 just from medical advances. Our ability to slow aging by then should push this number higher.

Continued biomedical research should empower medicine to prevent or cure 90 percent of all diseases. Although we almost certainly will have stopped the aging process by then, the conquest of most diseases will make its own contribution to the rise in life expectancy.

■ Health-conscious 35-year-olds can expect to live to 114.

■ Health-conscious 65-year-olds can expect to live to 114.

Those numbers, of course, are averages. Some health-conscious people may live only to 104, while others will live to 124. Still, extending life by medical advances, although essential, will reach a limit. Life expectancy will average around 115 until we can control the aging process.

7

What We Know About Aging

My diseases are an asthma and a dropsy,
and what is less curable, seventy-five.
—Samuel Johnson

Now, let's look at the most daunting barrier of all—aging. Beyond 100, after you have triumphed over cardiovascular disease, cancer, stroke, lung disease, accidents, diabetes, pneumonia, and a dozen other diseases, you face the final barrier. It is higher than any of the others you have faced. Yet there is a bright side. If aging is the final barrier, then its conquest will take you to the unthinkable. It will open the road not only for you to live 300 years but also to an indefinite life span, limited only by accidents or unexpected diseases. Hence, we are looking at bigger stakes than landing on the moon or splitting the atom. We are looking into the awesome portals of Shangri-la and changing the course of human history.

Yet, to a scientist, the conquest of aging is no different than the conquest of any disease. The first step is to define what it is and understand its nature. Let's see what we know about this deadly scourge we all share. One of my molecular biology students once said, "I can't define aging, but I sure as hell know it when I see it." Actually, aging is a set of programmed deteriorative processes that unfailingly lead to death. All too frequently, we think of aging in terms of appearance. Like my student, we feel that we know it when we see it. We see its power when we compare a 20-year-old with an 80-year-old. There's a big difference in appearance. The younger person also will perform better physically than the older one. But mentally the older person, unless a victim of stroke or Alzheimer's, may shock the 20-year-old. Elderly scientists and other scholars can outwit most of today's teenagers with ease. It's one of the indicators that aging causes different body functions to deteriorate at different rates. Still, aging has a profound overall effect.

Some qualities that make our 80-year-old appear aged are gray or white hair, wrinkled face, a slow, unsteady gait, and occasionally a glum outlook. But you can change surface features. You can change hair color from gray or white to brown, black, blond, or whatever color you want. A plastic surgeon can eliminate wrinkles with surgery and Retin-A. Exercise can improve health and vigor. In addition, you must "think young" because we know how potent the mind is in controlling the body. As a result, you may look 30 years younger. So much for knowing aging when we see it.

Many people take action against the external traits of age. More than half of American adults, men as well as women, color their hair. Many use retinoic creams to remove wrinkles and liver spots and give skin the smooth appearance of youth. This isn't vanity. A younger appearance moves you to a healthy, active life, improves your outlook, and aids your acceptance by society. This last factor is important because prejudice based on age in our society is as common as prejudice based on race or sex. As Dr. Robert Butler describes in his Pulitzer Prize-winning book *Why Survive? Being Old in America*, when you are older you are generally regarded as useless, senile, and rigid. Movie actors, business executives, members of congress, and even Presidents know that if you appear younger, prejudice tends to disappear. Little wonder that people color their hair and erase their wrinkles.

Some go further. Human growth hormone, a product of the pituitary gland, declines with age. As a result, lean body mass shrinks, fatty tissue grows, and skin thins. Lowered lean body mass is due to the deterioration of the muscles, liver, kidneys, spleen, skin, and bones as you age. Researchers have found that an injection of human growth hormone into elderly men causes a 9 percent rise in lean body mass, a 14 percent drop in fatty tissue, and a 7 percent increase in skin thickness. Livers, spleens, and muscles increase to sizes found in younger men. Evidence of how eager people are to stop aging is the sensation caused by reports of the action of human growth hormone. People have begged physicians for it. One group, ranging in age from 39 to 83, pays a Swiss clinic $5,400 every three months for injections. Maintaining a young appearance is important socially. But you are aging as fast as ever, so it is only a stopgap until we can halt the aging process. Let's see what we know about it.

The Characteristics of Aging

Every animal that has been studied carefully has a finite life span and shows similar deterioration with age. There are reports of sea anemones and fish with indefinite life spans, but they've not been studied enough to confirm the claims. Even plants show a surprising number of the same aging changes as animals. Watch the oldest leaves of a plant. The green color changes to yellow, then brown, as they die. If we measure what happens in the leaf cells, we find many of the same processes we see in cells of aging animals. Even bacteria may age under special conditions. Normally, they live forever if we give them nutrients to keep growing and reproducing. But if we give them plenty of nutrients and keep them from dividing, they rapidly develop many of the changes we see in the cells of aging animals. Within hours, they die.

Aging is a universal process, similar to other biological processes. It is no more mysterious, no more inevitable. The advantage of aging as a universal process is that we don't have to struggle initially with the problem of studying it in humans. We can study it in animals with shorter life spans. There are tiny worms that live only 5 days. Fruit flies live 3 months. Mice live 2 years, dogs 12, cats 20, and elephants 60. Humans (in Japan) average 79, and health-conscious humans average 100, but these are no records. Giant tortoises live 150 years. The famous bristlecone pines in California's Sierra Nevada live 4,000 years. Dr. Roy Walford reports in his book *Maximum Life Span* that creosote bushes in the Mojave Desert live 10,000 years. Clearly, different organisms age at different rates. Changes that take years in humans take months in mice. Changes that take weeks in mice, take days in fruit flies. The cells of all creatures have the ability to live for long times, since all cells are similar in structure and function. The need is to get cells to express their full potential to live. A characteristic of aging shared by all creatures is the deterioration of structure and function until an organism dies. Different activities fall at different rates. Some fall steeply, some decline slowly. The overall picture is one of deterioration.

The Effects of Aging

Instead of looking at hair color and wrinkles, let's look at changes that aging causes in the bodily processes essential to life. You may not realize how damaging aging is until you see what it does to them. Researchers have measured the effects of aging on hundreds of physiological and biochemical activities. In fact, much of the scientific literature on aging reports what aging does to every imaginable process in the body. As a result, we now have quite a clear picture.

Baltimore Longitudinal Study

An important source of information about human aging is the Baltimore Longitudinal Study by the U.S. National Institute on Aging. Located at the NIA's Gerontology Research Center (GRC) on the campus of Johns Hopkins University's Bayview Medical Center, the study has followed 650 volunteers since 1958. Each year, the volunteers spend two and a half days undergoing tests to determine what happens to the physical and mental functioning of their bodies as they age.

A major finding of the Baltimore Longitudinal Study is the variation in how fast each of us ages. We change at surprisingly different rates. You may have seen 80-year-olds who are vigorous and alert. They don't look or act 80. In contrast, there are people who age so rapidly they must retire at 62. They look and act 80. An extreme case is children stricken with progeria, a genetic disease that causes them to age so fast that they seldom reach their teens. Likewise, a particular function such as vision or hearing may change little in one person but decrease noticeably in another. In an annual report, the Baltimore Longitudinal Study sums up its findings: "NIA/GRC studies show a large variation in *how* individuals age. In observing a group of persons in their seventies, it is obvious that some are physically vigorous, mentally alert, and happy with their position in life. Others seem to slow down at much earlier ages." The changes are averages, with some people changing less and some changing more. Still, the Baltimore Longitudinal Study and researchers in medical schools, document an overall downward trend throughout life. By 85, functions have not dropped so far that they stop working, but they go down enough to impair your activity.

Let's look at measurements made by various researchers to see some things aging does to us.

Decline In Senses

When you think of decline due to age, impaired vision, hearing, and strength all come to mind. More people wear glasses as they get older, and you see more hearing aids. Figure 7-1 shows measurements that confirm your impression. Visual acuity (keenness of vision) drops steadily with age. At 80, vision averages 55 percent of what it was at age 20. At the same time, the frequency of cataracts rises. Loss of hearing parallels the loss of vision. At eighty, it averages 65 percent of its ability at age 20.

Figure 7-1. Decline in Senses

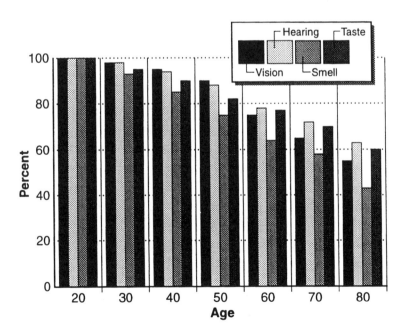

Not as well known is the decline in other senses. Taste, at age 80, is 60 percent as sensitive as at age 20. (Does that apply to red curry at a Thai restaurant?) The ability to detect and identify four odors (coffee, almond, peppermint, and coal tar) is only 43 percent as sharp at age 80 as at age 20. These are averages. Some people show no loss of taste or smell, while others lose one or the other sense entirely. A lower sense of taste and smell may be part of the reason old people often eat poorly.

Figure 7-1 shows the decline in four senses. But the picture is not all dark. Glasses and cataract surgery can restore most vision. Hearing aids are good at restoring hearing. We can't do anything about the senses of smell or taste, but they do not disappear for most people at age 80. They merely fall an average of 50 percent.

Decreased Muscular Strength With Age

The strength of your muscles also declines with age. Figure 7-2 shows how age affects three abilities of muscles. Grip strength is the ability to squeeze something with your hand. It is high until you reach age 60, then it falls rapidly. By age 90, it is 30 percent of grip strength at age 20. The strength of the biceps and shoulder muscles declines the same way. It is easy to see why a 90-year-old can't arm wrestle a 20-year-old or beat him in a 100-yard dash. Even greater is the loss of work output, the ability to sustain a repetitive, physical effort over a long time. Figure 7-2 shows work output decreases earlier and faster to a level at 90 that is only 10 percent of what it was at 20. While troublesome, these declines aren't life threatening. Other functions degraded by aging are more serious.

Decreased Cardiovascular Function

In addition to the impaired cardiovascular activity from diseases, aging also lowers heart function in healthy people. Figure 7-3 shows the drop with age in cardiac output, a measure of the heart's ability to work. Between ages 20

Figure 7-2. Decline in Muscular Activity

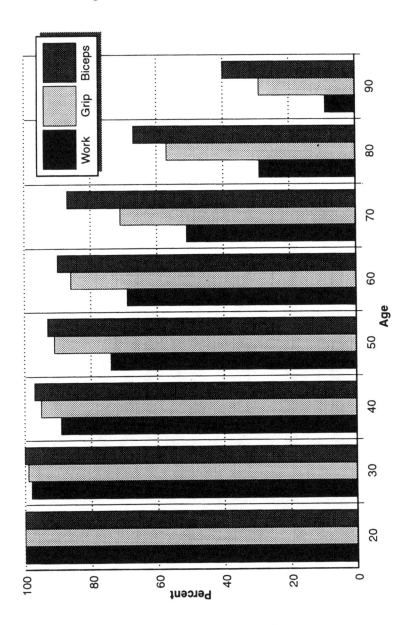

and 80, cardiac output falls 44 percent. Blood flow drops 50 percent. An abnormal electrocardiogram (ECG) indicates deviation from the heart's normal electrical pattern. Among the disorders causing it are partial blockage of the arteries feeding the heart, inflammation of the heart's membrane, heart failure, and abnormal heart rhythm. Abnormalities in the ECG are negligible in 20-year-olds but rise with age until they occur in 30 percent of 60-year-olds.

Figure 7-3. Decline in Heart Function

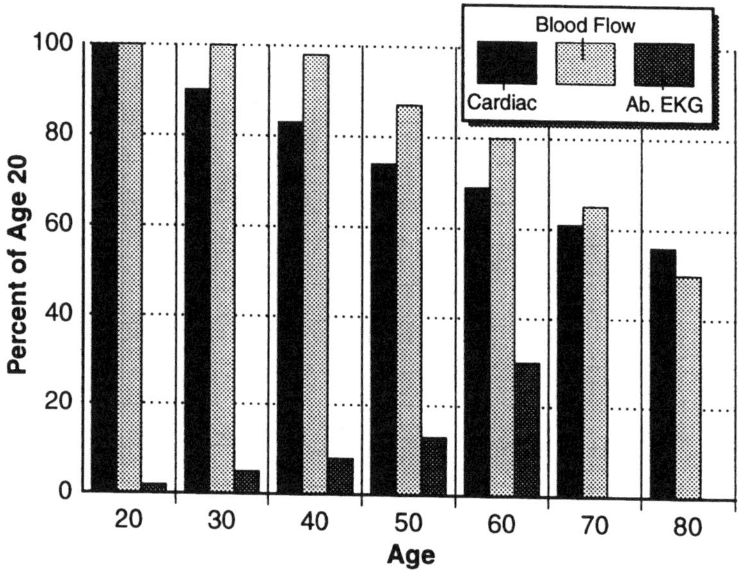

Decreased Organ Functions

Aging causes deterioration in the functions of your major organs. Figure 7-4 shows what happens to several as you age. Kidney function declines. Between age 20 and age 80, kidney function decreases 30 percent. The ability of the stomach to function also falls. Figure 7-4 shows the effect of age on acid secretion by the stomach in response to a test meal. Between ages 20 and 60, acid secretion drops almost 60 percent. Seeing that, you can understand why old adults often have digestive problems. The ability of the lungs to work efficiently declines. The effect of age on this function shows up in measurements of vital capacity, the air exhaled after a deep breath. Figure 7-4 shows that vital capacity in 80-year-olds is about half that of 20-year-olds. The amount of oxygen absorbed by the lungs falls steadily. By age 80, it's 56 percent of what it was at age 20. Hence, 80-year-olds gain only half the oxygen for their tissues as twenty year-olds.

The drops we have seen reduce many functions in 80-year-olds, but probably not enough to incapacitate them.

Figure 7-4. Decline in Organ Functions

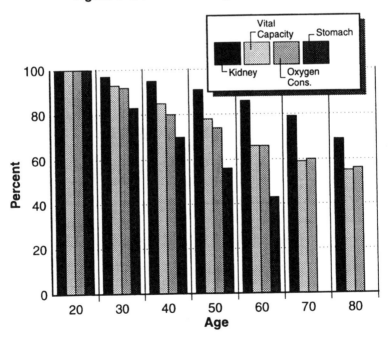

Growing numbers of 80-year-olds are healthy and active, so their organ systems must have ample reserve capacity. In contrast, look back at Figure 4-5, which shows how aging severely affects your immune system. The immune system, vital to defense against bacteria and other foreign invaders, also may have a protective function against cancer. The drop in immunity is one of the most perilous effects of aging.

Effects of the Decline in Functions on Maximum Life Span

Researchers have studied the effects of aging on hundreds of activities related to every operation of our bodies. By 85, the activities average about half of what we have at age 20.

The decreases in vital functions show us something important. Start with the trends that result in almost a 50 percent reduction in function between age 20 and age 80. Now, project the lines on downward at the same rate to ages past 100. If you extend the lines far enough, they intersect the age at which each function reaches zero. Those ages are the maximum attainable from curing diseases before the loss of that particular function kills us. Beyond those ages, further extension of life requires the control of aging.

Especially critical is immunity, which at age 100 is 10 percent of its level at age 20. Projecting its downward trend, immunity averages zero at 120. No wonder the maximum life span is currently 120-125. Since you can't live long without an immune system, anyone who lives past 120 probably has an immune system that has not decreased as fast as the average. Reduced immunity limits life to an earlier age (about 120) than any other process we know of. That is why vitamin E, multivitamins, and zinc to slow the decline of immunity are so important to longer life until we control aging.

Figure 7-5. Projections from Trends

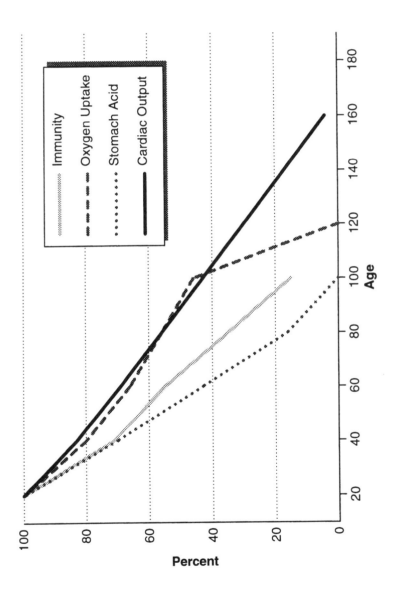

If we delay the drop in immunity, how else may aging limit life? Figure 7-5 shows what happens when we project trends in other bodily functions at the rates they decline between age 20 and age 80. Figure 7-5 shows that acid secretion by the stomach drops rapidly. Even if we reduce the rate a bit, it is zero, on average, by the time you reach 100. Whether maintaining an acid environment in the stomach is vital to life, its loss is still a problem for a 100-year-old. The acidic solution is essential for the digestive enzyme pepsin, which initially chops up the proteins you eat. But in the intestine there are other enzymes that cleave proteins completely. It is possible these enzymes digest proteins well enough to maintain the nutrition of 100-year-olds.

But other functions are vital. By age 80, cardiac output is 56 percent of its level at age 20. If we project this decrease to age 160, cardiac output drops almost to zero. Presumably, the body could not survive at some low cardiac output between ages 120 and 160, but 160 is certainly a maximum. That is a limit.

Thus, somewhere between the age of 120 and 160 (probably closer to 120), it will not matter how many diseases we prevent or cure. Unless we control aging, the conquest of diseases will be ineffective in extending life further. We probably can't live beyond 130 until we control aging.

The Road Ahead

In coming years, we will see reports of additional functions that decline in aging humans, rats, mice, fruit flies, and cultured cells. These data will give us a more-complete picture of the effects of aging on the body's activities. Most important will be findings of activities that decrease as fast as (or faster than) the immune system. Such declines could also limit life despite advances in medicine. But it is already clear that essentially everything deteriorates. That is the major theme of aging.

We must learn *how* aging causes all of these bodily functions to decrease. Since every function in the body occurs as a result of activities of the body's cells, we must probe inside those cells for the answer. That is the next step toward the control of aging and its awesome consequences.

8

The Causes Of Aging

"By far the most exciting, satisfying, and exhilarating time to be alive is the time in which we pass from ignorance to knowledge on these fundamental issues; the age when we begin in wonder and end in understanding. In all of the four-billion-year history of life on our planet, in all of the four-million-year history of the human family, there is only one generation privileged to live through that unique transitional moment: that generation is ours."
—Carl Sagan, Broca's Brain

To conquer aging, we must find its cause, and this means searching inside our cells. The reward, as medicine overcomes more and more diseases, is ever-longer life leading to an indefinite life span. The stakes are immense, so the search is as momentous as anything in history.

We often forget that the cells comprising us are wondrous systems. They import food and convert it to energy and materials for their activities. They repair and replace their parts. They manufacture substances and export them to other cells. They even construct exact duplicates of themselves.

But understanding cells is frequently regarded as improbable because of their complexity. Biology courses often depict a cell as a square thing on a yellowed chart hanging from the blackboard. In the center is a circular nucleus, and surrounding it is cytoplasm, which looks like London from ten thousand feet on a foggy day. You get the notion that the cell is infinitely complex—something we can never understand.

The Structure Of Our Cells

Infinitely complex? A cell doesn't have nearly as many parts as the Apollo/Saturn vehicle that took astronauts to the moon. NASA's computers cataloged its thousands of components. We are doing the same for every component of a cell.

Rather than foggy chaos, a cell is a defined structure. Think of it as a factory. Inside the factory are departments with distinct functions. The departments in a cell are its *organelles*. Each performs its share of the activities that cause us to live.

For the sake of clarity, we depict cells, as in Figure 8-1, to be roomy places where organelles have lots of space to go about their business. Actually, the interior of a cell is more like a crowded sweatshop, where organelles and proteins jostle and interfere with each other as they hustle about doing their jobs.

To understand what we know about the cause of aging, we must be familiar with the structure and inner working of a living cell. Hence, let's briefly visit the cell diagrammed in Figure 8-1, and look at its departments (organelles). The *cell membrane* is the factory wall, with gates to allow materials to enter and leave. *Microtubules* are structural girders. The *reticulum* aids structure and is the shipping department for material made by the cell. *Mitochondria* are power plants, converting food into energy for the cell's activities. *Lysosomes* are janitors, picking up and recycling worn-out parts. *Ribosomes* manufacture new parts. The *nucleus* controls it all, using directions recorded in its DNA.

Figure 8-1. Components of a Cell

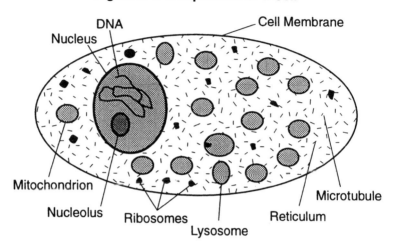

Organelles are composed of hundreds of different kinds of *proteins*, just as the departments in a factory are composed of concrete blocks for walls, and numerous pieces of machinery to do the factory's work. Many organelles also contain lipid (fatty material), and two contain DNA, but organelles are primarily made of proteins.

Proteins are the basis of life. Without them, you wouldn't be here, since you are made of proteins. Some proteins are structural, the bricks that hold us together, but most are microscopic machines that work with astounding speed and accuracy. Other proteins send and receive messages at the cell's surface or control the operation of groups of proteins. No machine built by man rivals the ability of a protein.

We can separate the cell's proteins from each other on a big, Jello-like slab of polyacrylamide gel, which has the ability to separate proteins in one direction according to tiny differences in electrical charge, and in a perpendicular direction according to differences in size. This separates the approximately 2000 different proteins in a cell, where they speckle across the slab like a swarm of dots on a sheet of paper. All the mystery of life is laid out before you on the slab, because the result of these 2000 proteins working together is the marvel we call life. Some people think life is a mystic process beyond understanding. That is non-sense. Life is the result of cooperative action of the cell's proteins.

The minimum number of proteins needed to produce life is astonishingly small. The tiny bacterium, *Mycoplasma*, needs only 470 different proteins in order to grow, divide, and wiggle under the microscope, completely alive. If 470 seems a lot, think of a flat box with 22 compartments per side. It would hold 484 proteins, more than the number needed for life.

Human cells contain more than four times the proteins of that tiny bacterium, but they are still not impossibly complex. We can separate their organelles from each other, then separate the proteins of each organelle. Approximate numbers are:

Cell membrane	140 proteins
Ribosome	78 proteins
Mitochondria	400 proteins
Lysosomes	100 proteins
Reticulum	150 proteins
Microtubules	4 proteins
Cell sap	532 proteins

A human cell has fewer parts than not only the Apollo-Saturn vehicle, but also the Space Shuttle and many machines you encounter daily. This allows researchers to search the cell for the cause of aging.

Effects of Aging on the Living Cell

The first place to look for the cause of aging is among the cell's organelles. Is one of the organelles altered or destroyed? Is something not operating properly? Has a malignant something formed inside the cell and is killing it? The first step toward an answer is to see whether aging harms any of the organelles.

Cell Membrane

Let's begin with the cell membrane. If you were shrunk to microscopic size, a cell membrane would look like something from *Alice in Wonderland*. It is a globule of fatty material that encloses the cell, like wall of a spherical building (think of the giant sphere at Disney's EPCOT) and studded with proteins like huge boulders embedded in stucco. Some membrane proteins are structural, but others have antenna-like projections to receive chemical signals. Transport proteins have a central orifice that opens and closes like the maw of an alien slug to slurp materials into the cell or spew them out.

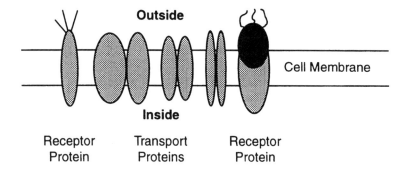

Outside

Cell Membrane

Inside

Receptor Protein   Transport Proteins   Receptor Protein

But the eroded membrane of an old cell looks like the exterior of an abandoned building in the slums. Receptors are missing, and transport proteins are damaged or missing. The cell does not respond well to changing conditions and

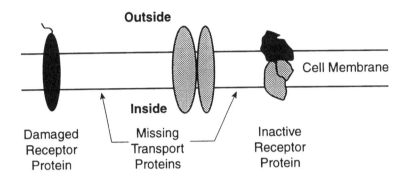

is slow at transport materials. Thus, aging causes massive deterioration of the cell membrane.

Mitochondria

Scattered through the cell, its power plants, the mitochondria, look like striped dirigibles, but they can twist into odd shapes. They have an outer membrane, a knobby, inner membrane that fills most of the organelle, and proteins between the membranes.

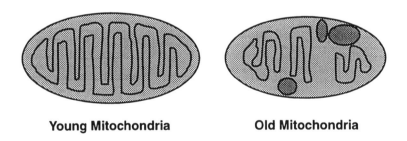

Young Mitochondria   **Old Mitochondria**

Aging causes both degradation and loss of mitochondria. Their organized structure becomes loose, and the inner membrane breaks up. Fluid-filled sacs appear inside. The number of mitochondria in each cell declines. Figure 8-2 shows how you lose mitochondria as you age. They begin to go at fifty. By seventy, a third of them are gone,

Figure 8-2. Drop in Human Mitochondria

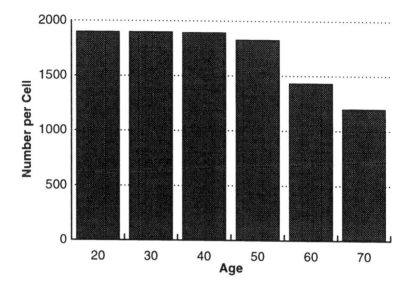

and those remaining are increasingly eroded and filled with fluid.

The visible damage and loss of mitochondria is reflected in impaired ability to convert foods into energy. If anything, it is even more sensitive to aging than mitochondrial structure, and you lose it steadily with age. In some animals, as much as 70 percent of the ability to produce useful energy is lost in old age.

Thus, the cell membrane is not the only organelle harmed by aging. It causes massive derangement and loss of the cell's power plants.

Lysosomes

These recyclers are as large as mitochondria, but without the convoluted, inner membrane. When first formed, lysosomes are circular, but can become amoeba-like and slither through the cell like The Blob to engulf worn or damaged proteins. Inside the lysosomes, proteins digest absorbed matter for recycling.

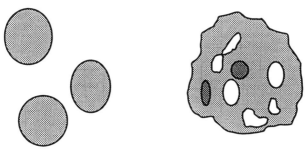

Young Lysosmes   **Old Lysosmes**

In young cells, small, circular lysosomes predominate. They do their job, then are replaced by new lysosomes. But in old cells, lysosomes are not replaced, and their proteins lose the ability to digest worn proteins that the lysosomes engulf. The old cell fills with enlarged lysosomes stuffed with undigested material. This is due to the aging process causing old cells to lose their ability to make new lysosomes.

Reticulum

As its name implies, the reticulum is a tubular network running throughout the cell, supporting the cell's structure, synthesizing materials, and exporting proteins or other materials to other cells. In young cells, the network is extensive. Aging causes cells to fail to replace the proteins comprising the network. The network shrinks, and its activity falls.

Ribosomes

Young cells have hordes of tiny ribosomes manufacturing new proteins. Since the cell's proteins constantly wear out and must be replaced, ribosomes are immensely important. Ribosomes have two-parts, a large unit and small unit fitting together. The units regularly separate, then clamp down on a thread-like pattern for a new protein. As the pattern runs through it, the ribosome makes the prescribed protein.

But if we look at an old cell, we see an astonishing loss of ribosomes. Whether in mice or men, at least half of the cells' ribosomes are missing by the time they reach old age. Aging causes a failure to replace worn-out ribosomes.

Cell Sap

Surrounding the organelles in cells is a clear fluid containing more than 500 different proteins. The proteins are of all sorts that perform essential steps in the cell's activities. With age, many of them increasingly lose activity, and aging causes a failure to replace them.

Nucleus

The control center and biggest structure in a cell is its nucleus. It is a sphere surrounded by a *nuclear membrane.* The membrane's most-visible features are big pores—actually gates. They are needed because ribosomes form in the nucleus. A dense body, the *nucleolus,* makes the framework for ribosome structure. The seventy-eight ribosome proteins travel into the nucleus and aggregate around the framework to form ribosomes. The new ribosomes must get out of the nucleus, hence big gates for them to pass through.

Chromatin harbors the cell's precious, yard-long strand of DNA, containing the genes for every protein in your body. Chromatin proteins protect the DNA and regulatory proteins control its genes. Surrounding the chromatin and nucleolus is a *nucleoplasm* of many proteins that aid the nucleus in its operation.

In old cells, the nucleus becomes lobed, eroded, and disorganized. Pockets of fluid often form, and granular bodies appear. It appears to be deteriorating. It may be that

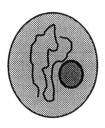 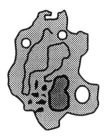

Young Nucleus   **Old Nucleus**

aging again causes a failure to replace worn-out proteins of the nucleus.

Thus, aging degrades the structures in your cells. Their neat forms become increasingly disorganized. Structures lose their tight appearance, becoming irregular and even fragmented. As organelles deteriorate, their ability to perform their tasks drops. Aging causes massive deterioration, even loss, of all parts of your cells. It obviously affects a common property of all parts of the cell in order to cause such widespread degradation.

Formation of Yellow Age Pigment

The first clue to one cause of aging came from the observations that aging cells, in addition to degraded structures, also form a bright-yellow substance. This *age pigment* accumulates in amazing amounts. Under the electron microscope, which doesn't show color, age pigment is visible as large, black granules filling cells.

Through the optical microscope, young cells have a healthy, pink color, but old cells show the fluorescent-yellow pallor of age pigment. The older you are, the more yellow your cells become. Accumulation of the yellow substance is so great that by the time you are ninety, 6 percent of your heart is age-pigment. This is similar to many of

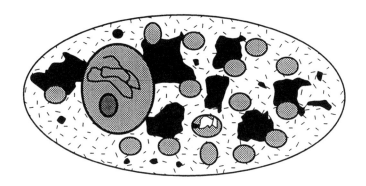

Age Pigment in a Cell

your organs, where age pigment deposits from the time you are twenty.

As startling as accumulation of age pigment is in most cells, its build-up in nerve cells is astounding. Figure 8-3 shows what happens in cells of your brain. The fraction of a nerve cell occupied by the nucleus drops from 26 percent at age thirty to 14 percent at ninety. The fraction that is cytoplasm falls from 38 percent to 13 percent. This is because the fraction occupied by age pigment squeezes down nucleus and cytoplasm as it expands from 36 percent to 73 percent. By ninety, age pigment takes up most of your brain!

Oxidation

Anything that accumulates to the extent that age pigment does in so many kinds of cells is a major consequence of aging. Thus, age pigment, along with deterioration of cell structures, is an important lead to one cause of aging.

But to pursue this lead, researchers could not use humans as experimental subjects. It is unthinkable to feed untested drugs to humans or subject them to other untested procedures. Aside from ethical reasons, there are also the

Figure 8-3. Increase in Age Pigment

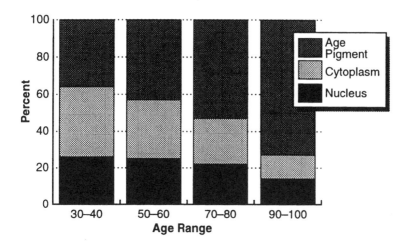

practical reasons that humans live too long and are difficult to study in large populations.

Fortunately, cells of other creatures are remarkably similar to human cells, and they change during aging in the same ways. The chief difference, which is an advantage, is they age faster than humans. We know that the shorter the life span, the faster the rate of aging. Hence, researchers employ a few, highly-useful helpers for research on aging.

Mice or rats have the same kinds of cells, the same organelles, and even similar proteins to those of humans. In the wild, they live only a few months, dying of diseases or predators. With clean environment, good nutrition, and humane care in the laboratory, the life expectancy of long-lived mice is 24 months, and rats 36 months. Still, the changes of aging in them are 30-40 times faster than in humans, so researchers can collect information quickly.

Fruit flies, the little fellows you see around bananas seem unlikely creatures to help find the cause of aging, but they are remarkably useful. Their cells have similar organelles and proteins to those in humans, and most of their cells are non-dividing, so they are all aging. Fruit flies only live three months, so they age with astonishing speed, and their cells show changes that take years in humans. We also probably know more about the genes of fruit flies than any other creature.

Caenorhabditis (see-no-rab-die-tis). This tiny round-worm, the size of a comma, has become incredibly useful to biomedical research. It contains many of the basic, human structures—muscles, nerves, blood vessels, digestive tract, and reproductive system. Yet, it is transparent, and each of its 959 cells is stunningly visible under a microscope.

An immense advance came when researchers found how to take individual cells from tissues and grow them in sterile, nutrient medium. Normal cells divide until they cover the bottom of the dish where they are growing. Cancer cells keep right on growing. The advantage of this technique is we can study human cells. Cells from a young person divide about fifty times, then die. Cells from an elderly person divide twenty or fewer times before dying. In both cases, near the end of the divisions, the cells exhibit *senescence*, where they undergo the same changes as aging cells in humans or animals.

What does research with these creatures tell us? The first thing we know is age pigment results from *oxidation* of fatty materials and proteins in the cell into a yellow mess. This is a life-long battle. You must have oxygen to oxidize foods to useful energy, but oxygen rusts your cells' building blocks to age pigment.

The second thing we know is, when you are young, your cells have special proteins that battle against oxidation. They don't protect cell structures totally, but they prevent rampant oxidation. But as you reach old age, these proteins dwindle and no longer protect the cell as well. By the time you are seventy, your cells will lose more than half of these proteins. This allows destructive oxidation to run wild in your cells to damage structures and produce age pigment.

The third thing we know is you can prevent accumulation of age pigment with *antioxidant* chemicals to combat oxidation. For example, when researchers fed mice a mixture of antioxidants (vitamin E, vitamin C, butylated hydroxytoluene, methionine, and selenium), it slowed formation of age pigment. Vitamins E and C, B-carotene, and selenium are good antioxidants. The drug, centrophenoxine, dramatically removes age pigment and prevents formation of more. A diet of fruits and vegetables, especially tomatoes, broccoli, and strawberries, reduces oxidation.

Some gerontologists suggested that oxidation is *the* cause of aging, but when researchers fed mice a daily dose of enough antioxidants to wipe out age pigment, it failed to extend life. Even big doses of antioxidants extend life of laboratory animals only 5-25 percent. Researchers also measured age pigment accumulation in two strains of fruit flies where one strain's life expectancy was a fourth of the other's. If oxidation is the only cause of aging, age pigment should form four-times faster in the short-lived strain. It doesn't. It accumulates at the same rate in both strains. Rather than the cause of aging, age pigment is likely a product of aging.

One cause of aging is this life-long oxidation that begins at birth and continues through life. In old age, when your protective proteins drop, oxidation increases and overwhelms your cells' ability to counteract it.

The drop in protective proteins is due to genes for these proteins switching off in old age, so they no longer supply patterns for the protective proteins. This effectively shuts off the supply of new, protective proteins.

But oxidation is not the only cause of aging. If it were, we would live forever merely by taking antioxidants, and that doesn't happen in laboratory animals or humans. In addition to oxidation, something else causes failure to re-place cell structures, resulting in massive deterioration and death.

Decreased Protein Synthesis

A momentous discovery about old age is that cells lose their ability to make new proteins. Loss of ability to manu-facture proteins may be the most important cause of aging. By the time you are eighty, different kinds of cells have lost 30-90 percent of their ability to make new proteins to replace worn-out ones.

The same loss in ability to make new proteins occurs in all other creatures. In our tiny friends, the fruit flies, old adults lose three-fourths of their ability to make proteins, and survival plummets. As protein synthesis continues to slide, the rest die. In laboratory rats, old adults lose as much as 80 percent of their ability to form proteins.

The drop results from a fall in formation of *all* proteins, rather than a halt in formation of some, but not others. Researchers have found the same fall in protein synthesis in old age in dozens of different animals and even in plants.

In addition to a decrease in protein-forming ability by the cell's ribosomes, synthesis of the dozen proteins made by mitochondria also drops with age. Protein synthesis by mitochondria of old mice is half that in young mice.

Let's look at how the drop in protein formation relates to how long a creature lives. Figure 8-4 shows it in long-lived mice, which average twenty-four months.

In the first twenty-one months of life, ability to make proteins declines about 15 percent. Then, in one month, between the ages of twenty-one and twenty-two months, it falls 45 percent more, for a total drop of 60 percent. As ability to make proteins continues to slide down, deteriora-tion soars and survival plummets.

Something occurs in that single month (possibly in a single week or single day) which has a catastrophic effect on the mouse's ability to live longer. The same occurs in other animals, from fruit flies to humans. There is little we could do as deadly as blocking our ability to make new proteins to replace worn ones. This is a major cause of aging.

**Figure 8-4. Protein Synthesis
and Survival in Long-Lived Mice**

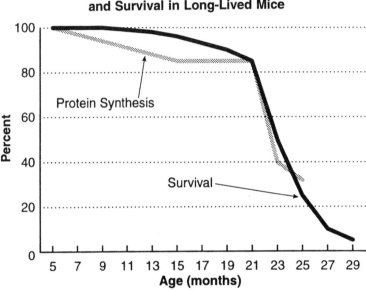

Serious consequences result from the loss of protein synthesis.

1. Deterioration of cellular structures as the protein-forming machinery fails to replace their component proteins.

2. Fall in activities of many proteins because they are replaced too slowly when they wear out. This impairs the ability of cells to operate.

3. Old cells become stuffed with worn-out proteins. In young cells, special proteins (proteases) break down worn

proteins for recycling into new proteins. But proteases also wear out. In young cells, other proteases break them down, but as we get old, failure of the protein synthesis machinery fails to replace worn-out proteases. For example, old mice have little more than one-tenth the protease activity of young mice. Worn-out proteases cannot break down other worn-out proteins, so worn proteins pile up in cells, like a garbage land-fill in a big city.

Because protein synthesis is so important, but so complex, researchers have scrutinized its fate in old cells. You recall that ribosomes make proteins. The process proceeds when a ribosome clamps onto a pattern for a protein. As the pattern feeds through the ribosome, it directs the ribosome to assemble building blocks into the new protein. To do this, the ribosome needs help from two, additional proteins, called "elongation proteins." When the ribosome reaches the end of the pattern, it releases the pattern and the new protein. The protein folds spontaneously into the shape it must have to become an efficient machine in your cell.

Old age curtails protein synthesis by retarding the assembly of building blocks into a new protein. It does this by switching off the genes for the elongation proteins and several proteins composing ribosomes. As with antioxidant proteins, the genes for elongation proteins and ribosome proteins almost stop producing patterns for these proteins.

Thus, when you reach an advanced age, the genes for key proteins "switch off." Evidence continues to pile up that this important happening triggers the catastrophic end of the aging process.

The Inability To Repair DNA

Age pigment and degraded cell structures jump out at us when we look at aging cells. But a clue to another, possible cause of aging comes from discoveries on what happens to your DNA as you age.

Throughout life, the DNA in your nuclei suffers continuous damage from radiation and chemicals. Fortunately, special proteins constantly repair the damage. But after twenty, they slowly decline. Then, when you reach old age, the proteins undergo a big drop. By eighty, you have less than half your ability to repair DNA. DNA breaks in a growing number of places. Since it stores the pattern for every protein needed for life, this is a calamity.

Among laboratory animals, when rats reach old age, they lose 70 percent of their ability to repair breaks in DNA. Mice, upon reaching old age, lose more than 80 percent of one repair protein and 95 percent of another.

Spectacular evidence that loss of DNA repair may be another cause of aging comes from discoveries on Werner's syndrome, an inherited disease where aging begins at 15-20, and quickly progresses to cause death at 30-40. At that age, victims have white hair, wrinkles, atherosclerosis, bone and muscle loss, and all features of a person over eighty. Researchers found the cause is lack of a protein that seems to help repair DNA. The protein lack results from a damaged gene for the protein.

The only other DNA in your cells is a tiny bit in mitochondria. This DNA provides patterns for a dozen, key proteins in mitochondria. In old age, it fares even worse than your nuclear DNA. In a spectacular case, when fruit flies reach old age, mitochondrial DNA disappears entirely. The age where it is gone is the fruit flies' maximum age. It makes sense. They can't live if they can't replace their worn-out power plants.

Thus, failure to repair breaks in DNA may be a third cause of aging. Repair ability declines throughout life, probably due to oxidation or declining replacement of worn-out repair proteins. Then, at an advanced age, a sharp loss of repair proteins, presumably from genes switching off, results in extensive damage to DNA which contributes to aging's massive deterioration of cells.

The Road Ahead

When researchers sought "the" cause of aging, they found instead that it has multiple causes. At present, there is evidence for three:

(1) Oxidation degrades our cells, attacking cell structures and individual proteins, much as it rusts metals (but produces age pigment instead of rust). It occurs throughout life, and accelerates in old age when antioxidant proteins diminish.

(2) Failure of protein synthesis has a domino effect as it reduces the supply of new proteins to replace those that wear out. This causes deterioration of cell structures and dwindling levels of proteins that do all manner of cellular activities, including protection from oxidative damage, repair of DNA, and recycling unfolded proteins. As a result, the cells degrade, causing the organism to wither until it dies.

(3) Failure to repair DNA causes the dramatic aging and death of young people with Werner's syndrome. Occasional failure of repair during adult life may cause slow deterioration by providing inaccurate patterns for proteins, but this accelerates in old age when the repair proteins vanish.

The three causes probably interrelate. For example, note in Figure 8-4 how protein synthesis declines slowly during the mouse's life before a massive collapse at twenty-one months. The slow decline could result from oxidative attack on ribosomes or other parts of the protein-making machinery.

Since the causes of aging have a devastating effect on life, the road ahead will be filled with efforts to stop them. Antioxidants, such as vitamin E or more powerful substances, in your diet may slow, or even stop, oxidation. Likewise, growth hormone partly restores protein synthesis, and you recall that growth hormone reverses some effects of aging in old men.

But the greatest ravages of aging result from dramatic losses in old age of antioxidant proteins, DNA repair proteins, and proteins in the protein-making machinery. This is due to the genes for these proteins switching off and no longer producing patterns for ribosomes to produce new proteins to replace ones worn out. Switched-off genes are the ultimate cause of aging.

Tracking down this underlying cause is a challenge, but its consequences are enormous. For example, if we find how to switch on the genes needed for your protein synthesis machinery, we can restore protein formation to its level in young cells. This will replace all worn-out proteins with new proteins. The result will be young cells. If you have young cells, you will be physically-young, no matter what your age. Hence, control of genes that restores protein formation will not only stop your further deterioration, but it also will return you to a physically-youthful state! It is better than Shangri-La, but it is the logical result of restoring protein formation to its original level.

We can draw an analogy with an automobile. When new (young), it runs well. As time passes, parts wear out and fail. If we do not replace them, the car shows wear and tear, and inevitably stops running. (The life expectancy of U.S. cars is seven years.) But if we continue to replace the car's parts, it will run forever. *The Guiness Book of World Records* documents a car that has kept in operation since 1922. By replacing parts, the car becomes "immortal."

Hence, a goal of research is to find what switches off genes for the protein-making machinery, DNA repair, and antioxidant proteins, and how to switch them on. Research has far to go on this knotty problem, but it is making astonishing progress. Researchers are also using knowledge of aging to produce substances to slow the process. But while they do, work on the genes that cause aging continues. It will make you physically-youthful, and if you avoid diseases and accidents, it will extend your life indefinitely.

9

The Search For Shangri-La

There is reason to hope that I will enter
lamahood with such prospects as Shangri-la has made
possible. In years, perhaps another century or more.
—Chang, in James Hilton's *Lost Horizon*

Now that we know something about what causes aging, let's see how researchers are using this knowledge to extend life. There are two ways to do it. You can wait until we can control the genes that cause aging, giving you an unlimited life span. You also can try to find something to extend your life a limited amount, say 30-50 years, by slowing aging. We will talk about this second approach first, then go for the ultimate in the next chapter.

Since the description of the Tree of Life in Genesis and the 5,000-year-old legend of Gilgamesh's search for immortality, people have sought a way to stop aging. Today, this desire finds millions taking all manner of substances claimed to extend life. Many take a daily 400-800 units of vitamin E, 1000 mg of vitamin C, 100 milligram of selenium, and 25,000 units of beta-carotene. This is understandable because these antioxidants may extend life by preventing cancer, cardiovascular disease, infections, and wear and tear in cells. Inclusion of plenty of fruits and vegetables in

your diet provides additional antioxidants, including ly-
copene from tomatoes (twice as powerful as beta-carotene)
and other potent ones from broccoli and related vegetables.

But some people take huge doses of vitamins and
amino acids in the hope of extending life. This is unwise,
since there is no evidence they are effective. It is also
dangerous because excessive amounts of some vitamins
and amino acids are toxic. For example, too much vitamin
A turns you an unearthly shade of orange and destroys
your liver. Others don't stop there. They take herbal pills
from health food stores. Coenzyme Q is popular. So is
"cleaning your blood" with EDTA, a process called chela-
tion therapy. Garlic, Ginkgo, and Ginseng are big. Gerovital
(essentially the anesthetic procaine) has its followers. Some
take superoxide dismutase, despite the fact that it is a
protein destroyed in the stomach. So it goes.

Except for antioxidants, the trouble with all this dosing
is there is no body of verified evidence that these substances extend life. There are no well-designed studies on
thousands, even hundreds, of people. There are no reports
in the *New England Journal of Medicine* or other respected
journals, reviewed by tough critics, that the substances are
effective. People are dosing themselves with things before
we have evidence about them. At best, they are a waste of
money. At worst, they are harmful. This is reminiscent of
laetrile, an extract from peach pits claimed to cure cancer.
The U.S. Food and Drug Administration banned it because
it saw no evidence that laetrile cures cancer. But cancer
victims, desperate for cures, traveled to Mexico to purchase
laetrile. Finally, a careful study showed laetrile has no effect on cancer. In fact, it contains cyanide, a poison. Since
then, we have heard little about laetrile. We need the same
kind of careful study of substances that are claimed to stop
aging. If companies making the claims are not simply trying
to swindle people, they should sponsor research aimed at

finding whether the substances are effective. It is always possible that some will be surprisingly useful.

In addition to garlic, ginkgo, and the rest, two substances have captured widespread interest due to extravagant claims about their powers.

Dehydroepiandrosterone (DHEA) is the chief product of our adrenal glands. Although its function is unknown, the quantity produced suggests it may play a key role in our bodies. It also occurs in large amounts in the Mexican yam. DHEA is interesting because its level in the blood drops with age, from 0.48 micrograms/milliliter at age 20 to 0.02 micrograms/milliliter at age 80. Anything falling that much makes you wonder about the effect of the drop. One answer is that people with heart disease have low levels of DHEA, and women with low levels of DHEA have a higher incidence of breast cancer. Thus, some gerontologists have proposed that the loss of DHEA may be a cause of aging, with a consequent rise in cardiovascular diseases and cancer. To test this, researchers compared twenty-four untreated mice with twenty-six mice given DHEA three times per week. After 9 months, more than half of the untreated mice had breast cancer. But none of the mice taking DHEA developed cancer. In a larger study, 27 percent of untreated mice developed breast cancer, but only 11 percent of mice fed DHEA. In mice exposed to the cancer inducer DMBA, 61 percent developed lung cancer, compared to 30 percent in DHEA-fed mice. DHEA may extend life by preventing cancer or cardiovascular disease, but there is no evidence it slows aging. Despite this, DHEA nevertheless has been promoted as a means to prevent aging. The Internet is full of pleas for sources where people can purchase it. But DHEA is only a tantalizing possibility.

Melatonin is a product of the pineal gland. Its level is highest during sleep. People with insomnia have low levels of melatonin in their blood. Doses of 0.3-2.0 milligrams per day help prevent insomnia. Doses of 5 milligrams per day reduce jet lag. Although researchers have found melatonin increases the survival of mice 20-25 percent, there is no evidence it retards aging. Despite this, melatonin has been ballyhooed as an anti-aging panacea. The Internet also hums with people, especially young ones, seeking the proper dose to keep them from aging.

The popularity of these products illustrates a yearning for a pill you can swallow to live longer. Thousands of people do all sorts of things hoping to extend life. Magazines devoted to health, health foods, and alternative medicine have advertisements for masses of life-extending pills. We see this yearning in the popularity of alleged anti-aging diets and even meditation as ways to stop aging, although there is no evidence any of them is effective.

The Search for Substances that Slow Aging

While people have spent millions on unproven anti-aging preparations, researchers have progressed in the search for drugs that diminish the effects of aging or even slow the aging process. Their quest is a good example of the exemplary and the unfortunate in research.

An obvious approach to finding substances that may affect aging is to discover what happens in aging cells and to try to block it. We know aging causes (1) the oxidation that degrades organelles and forms a yellow pigment, (2) a failure to repair DNA, (3) a failure to degrade inactive proteins, (4) the loss of activity of proteins, and (5) a drop in the formation of new proteins. If we find ways to retard any of these, we may curtail some effects of aging or slow the aging process. In examining progress, we must distinguish between effects on *life expectancy* (or survival) and effects on *maximum life span*. A substance may raise life expectancy by preventing diseases without affecting aging. But aging limits the maximum life span, even if we cure all diseases. Thus, if something boosts maximum life span markedly, it probably does so by slowing aging.

Experiments with laboratory animals have uncovered drugs that slow the aging process. Several are so promising that they warrant more study. Researchers are discovering more. We are on the road to slowing aging.

Antioxidants

Logical candidates to extend life are antioxidants. We know that oxidative damage to cells (especially aging cells) degrades cell structures, damages DNA, and piles up yellow age pigment. Oxidation appears to be one of the causes of aging. Chemically, antioxidants are reducing agents, the opposite of oxidizing agents. They are able to counteract oxidizing agents. But not all reducing agents can be used in cells. Some of the most powerful (such as sodium borohydride) are toxic, but many are not.

Vitamin E

A reasonable antioxidant for humans is vitamin E. It is a natural antioxidant in cells and is nontoxic. We know that it raises immune activity and lowers the incidence of cancers in laboratory animals. When researchers added 0.25 percent vitamin E to mouse food, it increased their survival 6 percent, but had no effect on maximum life span. That's a high level of vitamin E compared to what we humans take daily. Even at that level, it may hike life expectancy but probably does not slow aging. A clue to how vitamin E extends life comes from the discovery that mice fed this high level of vitamin E have only one-third of the cancer of untreated mice. This agrees with evidence in chapter 3 that vitamin E prevents some kinds of cancer.

If it has the same effect on humans as it has on mice, it could raise a 35-year-old's life expectancy from 78 to 82. Life expectancy of a health-conscious 35-year-old would jump from 101 to 106. This isn't much, but a jump in life expectancy of 6 years from swallowing a daily capsule is an easy way to extend life. We need to know more about the life-extending effects of vitamin E. Researchers should determine whether 400-800 daily units of vitamin E will boost life expectancy in humans.

A 6 percent boost in life expectancy may be the maximum effect of vitamin E, or the amount of vitamin E getting into cells may be too small to be more effective. We can overcome the difficulty of not knowing how much vitamin E the blood transports to cells by testing its effect on creatures that absorb it directly into their cells. In the tiny worm *Caenorhabditis*, vitamin E boosts survival 15 percent and maximum life span 12 percent. In rotifers, microscopic, free-swimming animals, it hikes survival 17 percent and maximum life span 14 percent.

Mercaptoethylamine

The possibility that antioxidants may prolong life was first realized by Dr. Denham Harman at the University of Nebraska Medical School. He began with five antioxidants: vitamin C, diethyldiaminodisulfide (DDD), cysteine, mercaptoethanol, and mercaptoethylamine (MEA). MEA was developed during the atom bomb scares in the 1950s to try to prevent deaths from radiation.

To test their effects, he added each to the food of short-lived mice of a strain called AKR. They live, on average, only 7.5 months. These mice offer the advantage of seeing quickly any effect of an antioxidant. The disadvantage is their short life, for they usually die early of leukemia. Neither vitamin C nor mercaptoethanol increased survival. But 0.5 percent MEA boosted it 9 percent. One percent MEA increased it 40 percent. A 40 percent jump in survival is exciting. The difference between the two levels of MEA shows why we must know the effect of a range of dosages. Another dosage may be even more effective. In addition to finding the effects of many concentrations, we also need to know whether the effect of MEA is universal. Feeding 1 percent MEA to C3H mice, a strain that often dies of mammary cancer, causes them to survive 26 percent longer. Feeding it to LAF mice, a medium-lived strain that doesn't get much cancer, raises survival 12 percent.

None of the antioxidants raised their maximum life span, so they had no effect on aging. MEA, like vitamin E, may increase survival by preventing cancer. The more prone the mice were to cancer, the more MEA raised their survival. We don't know whether dietary MEA would lower cancer incidence in humans or whether an effect on human cancer would be enough to raise life expectancy. Still, Harman's findings with MEA blazed a trail toward more effective antioxidants by showing they have the ability to increase life expectancy.

Butylated Hydroxytoluene

A popular antioxidant is butylated hydroxytoluene (BHT). Many food companies add it as a preservative to a variety of foods because it is effective. Low levels are not toxic.

BHT hikes the survival of medium-lived LAF mice 45 percent and medium-lived BALB mice 27 percent. These are impressive effects for an antioxidant. BHT requires more study in laboratory animals before we can consider whether it can raise the life expectancy of humans. Using drugs before thorough testing is unwise. Some people, after hearing claims (without evidence) that BHT stops herpes, foolishly took big doses. All they did was show that megadoses of BHT have nasty effects. Physicians treated patients who took two to six grams per day and suffered severe gastritis, weakness, nausea, dizziness, and even loss of consciousness. BHT raises the survival of mice but does not increase maximum life span, so it's doubtful it slows aging. But BHT provides more evidence that antioxidants may extend life expectancy.

Ethoxyquin

Another popular antioxidant, ethoxyquin (ETQ), is used not only for food preservation for humans but also to preserve animal and poultry feed. Agricultural scientists have noted that poultry on ETQ-treated feed retain fertility and egg-laying ability (youthful features) longer than poultry without it. Since ETQ is nontoxic and a powerful antioxidant, its potential effect on longevity is attractive.

ETQ increases the survival of medium-lived LAF mice an astonishing 75 percent. It raises the survival of medium-lived C3H mice 18 percent. Tumor incidence in these mice is low, so longer life may not be due to the reduction of cancer. Significantly, ETQ boosts maximum life span of C3H mice 29 percent, so it may slow that portion of aging due to oxidation. This is potentially important as a first step toward a drug to slow aging.

If ethoxyquin has the same effect on humans, it would raise life expectancy of a health-conscious 35-year-old to 118 and maximum life span to 155. That would be a stunning advance from a daily capsule. We need more laboratory studies before we can think of ETQ extending human life, including the effect of varied levels, its effect on the longevity of other animals, and its effect on the longevity of human cells in culture.

Thiazolidine Carboxylate

The possible usefulness of the antioxidant thiazolidine carboxylate (TCA) was first seen in fruit flies, where 0.2 percent in their food boosted survival 16 percent and maximum life span 17 percent. Tests of a series of TCA levels found the optimal dose was 0.3 percent, which hiked survival an impressive 77 percent and maximum life span 63 percent.

Using long-lived C57 mice with an average life of 28 months, researchers added 0.07 percent TCA to food beginning at 23 months. This is a tiny amount, and they began it very late in the lives of the mice. Despite the mice being so old (equivalent to 65-year-old people), 0.07 percent TCA still boosted survival 10 percent, from 28 to 31 months. TCA is the only antioxidant reported to extend the life of long-lived C57 mice. We need to know what other levels would do and what TCA would do if we were to feed it to mice throughout their lives. TCA also warrants more laboratory research on its action.

Despite all the hoopla in the media about the benefits of antioxidants, there hasn't been nearly the study of them that their potential warrants. Synthetic antioxidants show promising results in laboratory animals, but we have no badly needed evidence of whether they can extend human life, especially by slowing aging.

Even in laboratory animals, they display unexpected differences in activity. Some have no effect on survival. Others may raise survival by curbing cancer. Still others raise maximum life span, hinting at an effect on aging. Figure 9-1 compares MEA, BHT, ETQ, and TCA. MEA raises the survival of short-lived, cancer-prone mice but has little effect on medium-lived LAF mice. BHT boosts the survival of LAF mice more than MEA does and ups the survival of longer-lived BALB mice. ETQ raises the survival of LAF mice better than BHT but has less effect on longer-lived C3H mice. TCA, unlike the others, boosts the survival of long-lived mice.

Since antioxidants may extend life by preventing cancer, they deserve more study to find out whether they prevent specific cancers or prevent all cancers. They also may reduce cellular damage from oxidation, so we need to know more about their action. New antioxidants such as phenylbutylnitrone (PBN) may be more effective. Although still in the laboratory, antioxidants show promise as initial means to extend life and possibly to slow aging. We need thorough studies of ethoxyquin and similar antioxidants—first in animals, then if warranted, on markers of aging in

Figure 9-1. Life Extension by Antioxidants

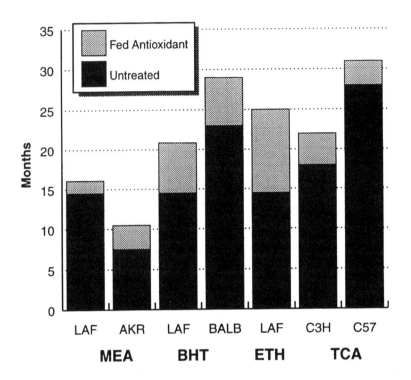

large groups of human volunteers. From this may come our first drugs to slow aging.

Calorie Restriction

The basis for another approach to life extension is the observation that animals with high rates of growth and metabolism have short lives. The slower the rates, the longer they live. Years ago, Drs. C.M. McCay, M.F. Crowell, and L.A. Maynard proposed a theory that slowing metabolism would extend life. To test it, they reduced the calories fed to Osborn-Mendel rats, a strain of laboratory rat especially used for nutritional study. When they lowered calories to 60 percent of what the rats usually eat, the result was startling. The rats lived an average of 41 percent longer.

Many studies confirm that cutting calories extends life in mice or rats. You can feed them less food or you can add cellulose to their diet. Even feeding 60 percent of the normal calories to pathogen-free rats has caused them to live 41 percent longer. Pathogen-free rats are longer lived than others, but calorie restriction has made them live even longer. More important, calorie restriction raises the maximum life span. Figure 9-2 shows that cutting calories raises

Figure 9-2. Calories and Life Span

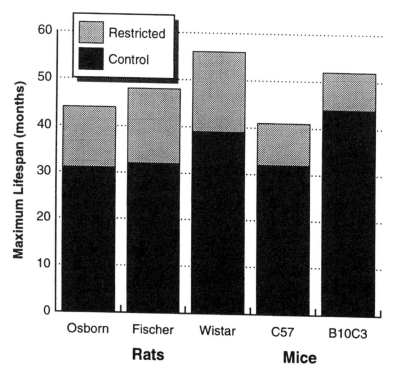

the maximum life span of various strains of rats and mice 18-50 percent. At least fifty reports confirm this and indicate it slows aging.

These effects on maximum life span are impressive because they tell us that aging is not a fixed process and that we can slow it by calorie restriction. Once we find how calorie restriction slows aging, we can find other ways to do it. To see how significant are the increases in maximum life span, if humans react the same, the life expectancy of 35-year-olds would rise from 78 to 109. The life expectancy of health-conscious 35-year-olds would rise from 100 to 141. Maximum life span would rise from 120 to 179 years.

In the *Bar Harbor* (Maine) *Times* of September 6, 1984, is a picture of a mouse at the Jackson Laboratories there. This mouse, on a restricted diet, lived twice her normal life expectancy. She was the first of a series of mice to live that long. In human terms, that is a life span of 160 years. More recently, Freddy, another calorie-restricted mouse, lived 1,742 days. In humans, that is a life span of almost 200 years.

Can calorie restriction extend human life? In his book *Maximum Life Span*, Dr. Roy Walford suggests it can raise your life expectancy to 120 years. He is likely correct, but you should consider several factors. First, calorie reduction extends life in at least seven strains of rats, seven strains of mice, and hamsters, but its effect is variable. The increase in survival ranges from 8 percent in long-lived C57 mice to 69 percent in Osborn-Mendel rats. The rise in maximum life span ranges from 18 percent in B10C3 mice to 50 percent in Fischer rats. Its effect on humans could be large or small. Second, studies by physiologist Ancel Keys during World War II on humans on low-calorie diets found the diets caused mental problems, lethargy, and increased disease. Of course, the diets were designed to study the effects of starvation. They were deficient in vitamins and minerals as well as calories. The provision of vitamins and minerals may prevent the difficulties seen in people on a starvation diet, but this requires further examination. Third, it is questionable if people will be thrilled about eating 40 percent less food each day. That is a permanent 1,200-1,400-calorie diet. Experience is that few people will stick to a diet with those scant calories in order to live 120 years or even 200 years.

One way to overcome the dislike of less food may be to replace part of the diet with cellulose or other inert material. Researchers at the National Institute on Aging did this with long-lived C57 mice. Antioxidants and calorie restriction showed little ability to extend the life of these mice, but replacing 50 percent of their food with cellulose extended survival an impressive 26 percent. Another possibility is a measured dose of a drug that will safely reduce the desire for food to 60 percent of usual intake. That may be better than cellulose.

Regardless of its effect on humans, calorie restriction is important because it shows we can slow aging. The way it operates is surprising. When we think of fewer calories, we think of life extension by elimination of obesity and cardiovascular disease. But calorie restriction goes far beyond that to slow the aging process as it hikes the maximum life span.

In laboratory animals, calorie restriction improves animals impressively. There is less heart disease. Degeneration of the heart slows. The incidence of tumors decreases. The decline in immunity slows. The decline in muscle slows. Kidney disease, a common cause of death in rats, occurs later in life and develops more slowly. By 27 months, one form of kidney disease occurred in 50 percent of rats eating freely. In contrast, no calorie-restricted rats had the disease, even at 36 months.

The possible cause of the improvement in health is as exciting as the event. We know that the synthesis of new proteins drops in old cells and is a major cause of aging.

Protein synthesis in the liver cells of rats fell 55 percent by the time the rats were 19 months old. But in calorie-restricted rats, protein synthesis in liver cells only dropped 9 percent. In testicular cells, protein synthesis dropped 40 percent, but in calorie-restricted rats it decreased not at all. In kidney cells, protein synthesis dropped 50 percent, but fell only 16 percent in calorie-restricted rats.

Thus, at least one effect—and perhaps the major effect—of calorie restriction is to slow the deadly drop in protein synthesis due to aging. Whether calorie restriction acts by affecting a hormone, a gene, or other factor, it does something basic to slow the drop in protein synthesis and to slow aging. Restricting calories may not be practical to prevent human aging, but it may lead to a means to slow it.

Anti-Aging Drugs

Although antioxidants have not yet shown a marked ability to slow aging, two drugs have. The first, centrophenoxine, has been prescribed by physicians in Europe for years to counteract aging. The second, deprenyl, is more effective than centrophenoxine and may be the forerunner of a series of even better drugs that will slow aging until we can control it.

Centrophenoxine

Chemically, centrophenoxine is dimethylaminoethyl-p-chlorophenoxyacetate, a synthetic relative of hormones that regulate growth, development, and even aging in plants. When plants age, their cells show the same deterioration as those in animals. In leaves, protein synthesis drops, cell structures degrade, and the loss of chlorophyll causes them to turn yellow before they die. French scientists found centrophenoxine delays the yellowing and the death of aging leaves. It is an anti-aging drug for plants.

Centrophenoxine became more interesting when researchers found that feeding it to old animals in the laboratory not only stopped the formation of age pigment but also rid the animals of age pigment that had already accumulated. Researchers found it had the same ability in a variety of animals. It probably does the same in humans. Its removal of age pigment caused researchers to wonder whether it retards aging in animals as well as plants. To test it, they added 0.03 percent centrophenoxine to the drinking water of mice, starting when they were 9 months old. Even this tiny amount raised survival 27 percent. More important, it boosted maximum life span a satisfying 27 percent, indicating that it delays aging. If it has the same effect in humans, it would raise life expectancy of health-conscious 35-year-olds to 127 and the maximum life span to 152.

The possibility that centrophenoxine affects most animals comes from its ability to also extend the life of fruit flies, animals more distantly related to mice than mice are to humans. When researchers added 0.12 percent to their food, it hiked their survival 39 percent and the maximum life span 23 percent.

Thus, centrophenôxine shows promise as a drug to slow aging. There are several reasons why. Only 0.03 percent in drinking water raises the maximum life span of mice 27 percent. The actual amount is less because centrophenoxine breaks down quickly in water. At room temperature, half is gone in thirty-four minutes. Hence, the amount that raises the maximum lifespan is mostly what mice drink during the first hour after getting fresh water. This suggests that a tiny amount of centrophenoxine may be all that is needed to slow aging. A different dose may be more effective. Since researchers only studied a single dose, it would be remarkable to just happen to hit on the optimal one. Mice did not get centrophenoxine until they were 9 months old. Average survival of these mice was 18 months, so they got the drug for half their lives. Getting it for their entire life may raise the maximum life span further. Since centrophenoxine degrades in water, it might be more effective in dry food for mice, as it is for fruit flies.

Centrophenoxine passed a clinical trial in Germany without evidence of toxicity. It is sold by prescription to the elderly in Europe as Lucidril, Clofenoxine, Meclophenoxate, Helfergin, and ANP 235. It is reported to slow some effects of aging. Trials of its effect on human longevity are in progress in at least one European institute for research on aging.

Centrophenoxine is a candidate to retard aging in humans. But first we must know what dosage maximally increases life in laboratory animals, whether it would be more effective in food instead of water, its effect in different animals, and its effect on aging of human cells in culture.

Deprenyl

This well-known drug, which slows the onset of Parkinson's disease, is one of the most exciting possibilities to extend life. Starting when you are 45, the level of dopamine, an essential transmitter of signals in your brain, declines an average of 13 percent every 10 years. Parkinson's disease develops when the dopamine level falls to about 30 percent of its initial level. Since it usually doesn't reach 35 percent until you are 95, most people are unaffected. But as more people live past 100, Parkinson's disease could become a growing problem.

Some people lose more than 13 percent of dopamine every 10 years, so Parkinson's appears earlier. The standard treatment for Parkinson's disease is dihydroxyphenylalanine (DOPA). Unfortunately, after you take DOPA for a time, it loses its proficiency against Parkinson's disease. Deprenyl slows the decline in dopamine, delays the onset of Parkinson's, and extends the period before DOPA is needed. In 1985, researchers noted that elderly Parkinson's patients taking DOPA plus deprenyl lived an average of 18 months longer than patients taking DOPA alone. This was a marked effect for a drug that people, already very old, had taken for only a short time. It suggests that deprenyl may increase longevity.

To test deprenyl, researchers compared the survival of rats given deprenyl with that of untreated rats. Treatment began when the rats were 104 weeks old, equivalent to 55-year-old humans. Untreated rats lived an average of 147 weeks. The last untreated rat died at 164 weeks. Rats fed deprenyl did not begin to die until 2 months later! Thus, deprenyl-treated rats did not begin to die until well beyond the maximum life span of untreated rats. Deprenyl-treated rats lived an average of 196 weeks, a 33 percent rise in their survival. If we calculate increased survival from the time that deprenyl was first given to rats, it more than doubled their survival. The maximum life span for rats on deprenyl jumped from 164 weeks to 226 weeks, a 38 percent increase. If we calculate the increase in maximum life span from the time researchers first gave deprenyl to the rats, it also doubled the maximum life span. A second group of researchers began deprenyl treatment when rats were 18 months old. Deprenyl raised life expectancy 34 percent. The rats showed no weight loss, so deprenyl does not act by restricting calories. Other researchers gave deprenyl to rats when they were very old. Despite the advanced age, deprenyl still boosted their survival and maximum life span roughly 16 percent.

Deprenyl had an unexpected effect when researchers gave it to mice that lacked an immune system and were therefore kept in a germ-free environment. Without the threat of bacterial infections, deprenyl raised their survival 60 percent and caused a nearly threefold increase in their maximum life span!

Deprenyl prolongs sexual activity, a youthful characteristic, in aging rats. In male rats, sexual activity had de-

clined by 104 weeks of age. At this point, a number of the
rats were given thrice-weekly deprenyl. Sexual activity in
untreated rats continued to drop to zero by 137 weeks.
Deprenyl restored full sexual activity in 97 percent of the
treated rats. These findings also support the idea that deprenyl slows aging.

If deprenyl acts similarly in humans, it would raise the
life expectancy of health- conscious 35-year-olds to 141. It
would also have the potential to raise the maximum life
span to 166 years. Based on its effect when first given to
rats, it might raise life expectancy to 160 years and the
maximum life span to 240 years.

Since deprenyl is the first drug to show a confirmed
ability to delay aging significantly in laboratory animals, we
must know more about it. What happens when we give it
to animals at earlier ages? What is the optimal dose? Does
it act the same in different strains of mice or rats? Is its
anti-aging effect related to dopamine, or does it have a
different effect on aging? Does it slow the aging of human
cells in culture?

What is its effect on humans? From exhaustive testing
for approval by the U.S. Food and Drug Administration,
deprenyl is safe for humans. We need a comparison of the
rate of aging of large numbers of persons who take deprenyl with those who do not. If more studies confirm its
effectiveness in extending the life of animals and raising
the longevity of people, deprenyl may dramatically slow
your aging.

Studies On Humans

If deprenyl, centrophenoxine, or an antioxidant shows
promise in further studies with laboratory animals, how do
we study the effects of each on human longevity? It is
impractical to do the usual kinds of longevity studies on
humans. It would, after all, take a lifetime. Instead, we
measure the rate of aging. The best measurements are

those used by the National Institute on Aging's Baltimore Longitudinal Study. If a drug slows these changes over a five- or ten-year period, it is probably slowing the aging process.

Another possibility is H-Scan, a computerized test machine. Looking like a video game, the instrument has a viewing screen, entry keys, earphones, a breathing tube, and attached diagnostic equipment. It uses fourteen tests of physiological characteristics of humans that change markedly during life. By following them yearly for several years, we can see measurable changes due to aging. We can also measure on a large population whether a substance slows aging. On promising drugs, five years should give an indication of the drug's ability. Ten years should give definitive information.

If preceded by extensive data from laboratory animals, tests of this sort will permit us to determine whether a drug will slow human aging. Although testing and approval for humans may take years, if researchers push vigorously we can have a drug to slow aging by 2015 or 2030. In the interim, it is likely that research with laboratory animals will find substances that are even more effective.

The Road Ahead

The effect of deprenyl and centrophenoxine on aging may be analogous to the way insulin acts on diabetics. It does not cure the disease. A cure may require gene therapy, but insulin controls diabetes and extends the life of diabetics. Likewise, the control of gene expression is probably needed to extend life indefinitely, but deprenyl and centrophenoxine may retard aging enough to increase longevity.

Figure 9-3 compares the amount that each increases longevity and the maximum lifespan. All have been effective in laboratory animals, but these probably are not optimal concentrations. Also, I have not seen reports of anyone

Figure 9-3. Drugs to Slow Aging

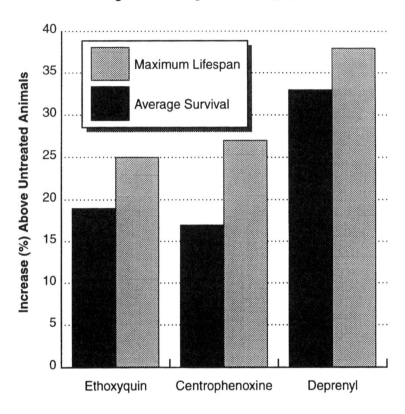

testing the effect of a combination (ethoxyquin plus deprenyl, for example) on life expectancy and maximum life span.

In view of the ability of ethoxyquin, deprenyl, and centrophenoxine to extend the life of laboratory animals, it is astonishing that more research has not been done to verify their effects on longevity. Deprenyl is especially exciting, since there has been so much confirmation of its action. But if any of the substances is as effective as reported, it has the potential to extend human life 20 to 40 years beyond that caused by the conquest of diseases. That is worth a big effort, as is the effort to find more effective drugs to slow aging. In the meantime, deprenyl may be our first drug to slow your aging effectively, extending the "youthful" portion of life 40-60 years. Alternatively, an antioxidant may be the first. It depends on which drugs undergo human testing first in the laboratories of universities or pharmaceutical companies. If these drugs are not the ones, another drug will be. Drugs to slow aging are coming, and the billions in income to someone will depend on which researchers work the fastest.

Deprenyl, centrophenoxine, ethoxyquin, and drugs still to be discovered are likely effective, but only interim, ways to slow aging. To stop aging completely, we almost certainly must control genes.

10

The Highway to Immortality

Gene splicing is the most awesome and powerful skill
acquired by man since the splitting of the atom.
  —John Naisbitt, *Megatrends*

Molecular biologists and genetic engineers are moving you toward an unlimited life. It is the ultimate, the unthinkable, but that is precisely where they are heading. What they are doing is also the most difficult to understand because you must know how genes act and how they are controlled. So hang on tight, and away we go.

By 2010 to 2030, deprenyl, antioxidants, or new drugs based on these or calorie restriction should raise the life expectancy of health-conscious persons to between 140 and 160 years. This is progress, but we saw in Chapter 8 that a major cause of the deterioration of aging—the collapse of protein manufacture—results from changes in the activity of genes. Drugs are unlikely to produce a 300-year (or indefinite) life unless they control the genes that cause aging. When we probe deeply into the aging process, we invariably find genes as the root cause of aging. As we identify and control these genes, we move as close to immortality as possible. The research problems are huge, and we have far to go, but the ultimate goal of people throughout history is coming into view.

Gene Control Of Longevity

We should have realized earlier that genes are the ultimate controls of longevity. Evidence for it has accumulated for years.

You inherit a tendency for long or short life from your parents. There is an ancient joke in gerontology: "If you want to live a long time, be sure to pick long-lived parents." (Gerontologists aren't noted for their wit.) The quip has a firm basis. Long-lived parents pass their longevity on to their children. For example, in 1918 Alexander Graham Bell, whose hobby was genealogy, studied the relationship of the lifespan of children to that of parents in 4,000 descendants of William Hyde. Bell found that the children of parents who died before age 60 lived only a little more than half as long as the children of parents who lived past 80. Even one long-lived parent raised the longevity of the offspring. Studies by insurance firms show the same thing. Among 50-year-old applicants whose parents are dead, the chance of an applicant dying early is almost 50 percent higher than if both parents are still alive. Parents give you genes for long or short life. Many factors shorten life, such as smoking, AIDS, or walking in front of a speeding truck. But accident or disease factors aside, long-lived parents have long-lived children. Short-lived parents have short-lived children. Heredity is due to genes. These observations are clear evidence of genes controlling longevity.

Females usually live longer than males. This is the case in humans and in almost all kinds of animals. In the pair of chromosomes specifying sex in humans, females have two X chromosomes (XX). Males have one X chromosome and one withered Y chromosome (XY). The two X chromosomes in females may give them twice the chance to have genes that raise longevity. Not having it may halve the chance for males, or genes in the Y chromosome may lower longevity. Whatever the case, it is more evidence that genes control longevity.

Different kinds of creatures with different genetic makeup have widely differing longevity. A housefly lives 30 days, a mouse lives 2 years, a human lives 100 years, and a bristlecone pine lives 4,000 years. The different ages result from differences in their genes.

In fruit flies, alteration of a single gene changes longevity. Fruit flies are remarkably useful in biomedical research because researchers have produced thousands of different mutants. These are flies with altered characteristics (such as white eyes instead of normal, red eyes) due to the damage to a single gene. In the black mutant, where the change in one gene causes the flies to be black instead of brown, the change also extends life 20 percent. But in the vestigial mutant, where a change in a different gene keeps wings from developing, the change drops the life span almost 70 percent. This again shows that genes control longevity.

Researchers can breed fruit flies for long life. If you breed old adults, you use creatures that possess youthful characteristics such as the ability to reproduce at an advanced age. This selects for genes giving increased longevity. Applying this concept, researchers have bred fruit flies for long life for twenty-five generations. (This shows why the short life span of fruit flies is useful. Think of the hundreds of years it would take to study twenty-five generations of humans.) As a result of breeding for long life, the average survival of the fruit flies rose from 38 days to 77 days, *doubling the creatures' lives.* Survival was longer than the maximum life span of the original generation. This longer life was due to postponed aging, extending the young adult phase of life. This is powerful evidence that genes control aging and longevity. It also shows that the control of genes can extend life spectacularly.

Some scientists have argued that genes can't control

aging because twins don't have identical life spans. For example, in one set, one died of cancer at 75, but the other was healthy at 93. But this doesn't rule out gene control of longevity. It simply says genes aren't the cause of death if a disease gets you first. Under 85, choice, chance, and environment affect whether you die of diseases or accidents. One twin might smoke and die first. Diseases and accidents govern longevity when we are younger, but genes increasingly govern it beyond 85.

Hereditary diseases, due to damaged genes, cause rapid aging. In Werner's syndrome, an inherited, defective gene causes young people to age rapidly. By age 40, they look like 80-year-olds and soon die. Even more extreme is progeria, in which a different defective gene causes rapid aging to begin about age 4. Victims usually die before they are 15 years old.

These observations leave no doubt that genes control longevity. Recognition of this fact is a major step toward longevity of 300 years or more. The task is to find out which genes govern longevity and how to control them.

Genes

Before we look at how genes may control longevity, let's review what genes are and how they operate. Life results from the action of more than 2,000 kinds of proteins working together in cells. Proteins wear out quickly and must be replaced. Genes store the patterns for the assembly of each protein.

Genes are segments of DNA, a long tape thinner than a spider's web. The best analogy for DNA and genes is to think of DNA as a videotape divided into segments that give instructions on how to build different things. One segment tells how to make a table, a second tells how to make a chair, a third tells how to make a cabinet, and so on. Genes are comparable to these segments containing instructions. Genes are the patterns for each protein responsible for life, but the cell can't take chances with its master tape of DNA. To make a protein, it copies the gene onto a short length of RNA, a tape similar to DNA. The process resembles transcribing a videotape, so molecular biologists call it *transcription*. The resulting tape contains instructions from one gene. Since the tape carries a message on how to make a protein, we call it messenger RNA (mRNA). Hence, the pattern stored in gene 1 becomes a working copy on mRNA 1.

The mRNA moves to a ribosome, which clamps onto one end of it. As the mRNA pattern feeds through it, the ribosome hooks building blocks together in the correct order to make the protein. Ribosomes will make any protein an mRNA directs. For example, a bacterial ribosome will make a human protein if we give it a human mRNA.

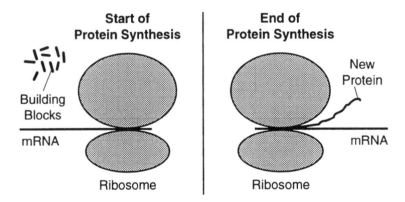

Start of
Protein Synthesis

Building
Blocks

mRNA

Ribosome

End of
Protein Synthesis

New
Protein

mRNA

Ribosome

You have more than 50,000 genes in the DNA in just one of your cells. They are all the genes needed to make another you. (When you discard a hangnail, you abort the potential to produce another human.) In each of your many different kinds of cells, only some 2,300 of the 50,000 genes supply patterns to make the 2,300 different proteins comprising that kind of cell. In skin cells, genes for skin proteins are transcribed but not genes for brain proteins. Molecular biologists refer to the genes actively being used to produce proteins as *switched on*. All other genes are *switched off*. This is important, because switching genes on or off controls longevity.

Control of each gene—whether it is switched on or off—resides in a segment of DNA next to the gene, called a promoter. There are three ways promoters control genes, and each is important for understanding how molecular biologists are moving you toward unlimited life.

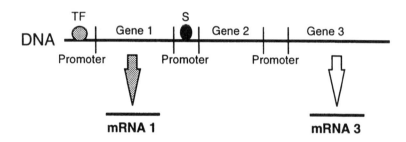

1. Genes can be fully switched on. *Transcription factors* (TF) are proteins that switch genes on by attaching to their promoters. Genes with transcription factors attached to their promoters operate at full speed. Transcription factors often control batteries of genes, sometimes hundreds. For example, in skin cells, a transcription factor might switch on all genes for skin proteins. In the diagram above, gene 1 has a transcription factor attached to its promoter, which causes its pattern to be copied at the maximum rate.

Genes can also operate slowly. You might think a gene without a transcription factor attached to its promoter is switched off, but most operate slowly in the absence of transcription factors. In the diagram, gene 3 is transcribing slowly in the absence of a transcription factor.

Genes can be switched off. *Suppressors* (S) are proteins

that switch genes off totally when they attach to the gene's promoter. They also often control whole batteries of genes. For example, suppressors switch off growth genes to prevent cancer. In the diagram, gene 2 is stopped by a suppressor attached to its promoter.

Growth, cell division, cellular activity, aging, and longevity all involve transcription factors or suppressors switching arrays of genes on or off. Their importance is obvious, and they are under intense study by researchers. As we learn more about their actions during aging, it moves us on toward the control of aging.

Changes In Gene Expression During Aging

Since genes control longevity, the first step toward an indefinite life span is to find out how many genes change to limit life. Once we know that, we need to know which genes change and whether they switch on or off. Barring death from disease or accidents, the control of these genes should extend life indefinitely. These questions are as important as any we can ask.

To get a picture of how gene expression changes with age, researchers have looked at the formation of all the proteins in young and old cells. Synthesis of proteins will decline because of the failure of the protein-making system. But if new proteins pop up, or others vanish, or still others change extremely, they indicate genes have switched on or off. Of the 500 proteins examined from human cells, aging caused 5 to climb and 4 to drop. Extrapolation to 2,300 proteins in human cells suggests that aging may involve changes in roughly 40 genes. Of the 1,000 proteins examined from mice, aging caused 5 to vanish, 9 to fall steeply, and 4 new proteins to appear, with 1 becoming abundant. Thus, 18 genes changed. Extrapolation to 2,300 proteins in mouse cells suggests that aging also may involve changes in some 40 genes.

The knowledge that aging is caused by directly chang-

ing the activity of a relatively small number of genes means
that we don't have to search thousands of genes for the
cause of aging. We should search for fewer than 50.

Changes In Specific Genes During Aging

Since the activities of so few genes change to cause
aging, the next step is to find out which genes change.
From the DNA → RNA → Protein pattern, we should be
able to detect a gene switched off by a big drop in its
mRNA or a gene switched on by a big rise in its mRNA.

Since the genes that change are likely to be for key
proteins in the operation of your cells, researchers searched
for large changes in the output of mRNAs for key proteins.
It didn't take long to find them. Aging causes an 85 percent
fall in mRNA for a protein that is a vital part of your
immune system. It caused 50-70 percent drops in mRNAs
for four other proteins critical to the operation of your cells.
Importantly, aging causes a 50 percent reduction in mRNAs
for three antioxidant proteins that are crucial defenses
against harmful oxidation in cells.

Equally important is the drop in mRNAs for proteins
that operate the protein-making machinery. Recall from
Chapter 8 that aging curtails the formation of new proteins
by halting the stage of protein manufacture where ribosomes assemble building blocks into proteins. To do this,
ribosomes need the help of two elongation proteins. Researchers have found that protein formation drops in old
age because of a loss of ribosomes and elongation proteins.
This must be a universal event in aging because researchers
have found it in creatures as unrelated as humans, mice,
and fruit flies. Researchers have found that ribosomes diminish because of a tenfold drop in the expression of
genes for six of the ribosome's proteins. They have found
the mRNAs for elongation proteins fall 50-90 percent. Direct
measurements of activity of the genes for elongation proteins show that they mostly switch off in old age. Phorbol

PMA, a chemical that causes genes to switch on, restores elongation proteins in old cells, confirming the genes were switched off. In simple creatures, damage to genes for elongation proteins causes enormous increases in life span. The damage may switch the genes on fully, with no control by genes that cause aging.

Hence, aging produces a cascade of events:

Ribosomal And Elongation Protein Genes Switch Off

↓

Elongation Proteins And Ribosomes Diminish

↓

Protein Synthesis Falls

↓

Replacement Of Worn-out Proteins Fades

↓

Your Cells Deteriorate And Die

Hence, discovery of what causes the reduced expression of these genes is truly a matter of life and death. Suppressors could switch off the genes, but a more likely cause is the loss of transcription factors. If a suppressor switched off ribosomal and elongation protein genes, protein synthesis would stop. But look again at Figure 8-4. Protein synthesis in old mice drops, then continues slowly. The same occurs in human cells and in our helpful friends, the fruit flies. The steep, but incomplete, drop is likely due to the loss of transcription factors. In fact, all the drops in gene expression that we have seen result in genes still active at 20-50 percent of their original rates. They seem due to a loss of transcription factors. This may be an important characteristic of aging. It is also a step toward finding the genes that cause aging.

Changes In Regulator Genes During Aging

You have learned that transcription factors are proteins that switch on batteries of genes. They are formed from patterns stored in *regulator genes*, which control anywhere from a few to hundreds of other genes. Researchers have found four well-known regulator genes that switch off during senescence in human cells. Each controls an array of genes for proteins in your cells. Researchers are testing whether aging switches off other regulator genes. Regardless of how many regulator genes aging switches off, researchers have taken an important step toward controlling aging. The cascade of aging becomes:

Switch Off Regulator Genes
↓
Curtail Key Genes By Loss Of Transcription Factors
↓
Cause Deterioration Of Cells And Death

Regulator genes, in turn, are controlled by genes that regulate regulators. As we find these, we move closer to the discovery of the genes that cause aging.

Genes Controlling Longevity

Now, we dig further into your DNA to find the genes causing aging. As we do, we reach the always-treacherous frontier of research.

Researchers have accumulated much evidence that senescence in human cells is due to a genetic program. Everything we see supports this evidence. Researchers also have found that the positive action of genes is needed for senescence to occur. This is important because it says an action must occur to switch off the regulator genes, thereby curtailing genes for protein formation and other activities. An obvious possibility is there are genes that cause aging and that some timing program switches them on after twenty-one months in long-lived laboratory mice or about 88 years in health-conscious humans.

The stunning fact is that researchers have begun to find genes that may cause aging in simple creatures. The first gene is age-1, a gene in the tiny worm *Caenorhabditis*. Because of its simple structure and small number of genes, this creature is hugely popular for biomedical research. The product of the age-1 gene limits life, since mutation (alteration) of the gene more than doubles the maximum life span. These longer-lived creatures with an altered age-1 gene have a high resistance to oxidation. The activities of two proteins that protect cells from oxidative damage are high compared with their activities in normal creatures. Apparently, the protein from the age-1 gene normally suppresses the production of these protective proteins.

Since the mutation of age-1 does not cause unlimited life, other genes must be involved in the control of the creature's life span. This is confirmed by the discovery of another gene, daf-2, which also controls longevity in *Caenorhabditis*. Mutation of daf-2 also more than doubles the lifespan, and the creatures remain active in old age. Damage to a third gene, daf-23, likewise doubles the life span.

Especially exciting was the result when a researcher damaged daf-2 and another gene, daf-12. She found it astonishingly *quadrupled their life span*. This suggests that a series of genes limits life. One genetic study suggests four or five genes control longevity in these creatures, while another suggests six. In any event, these may be the long-sought genes controlling longevity.

What happens if you alter various combinations of these genes, and what happens if you damage most or all of them? Will the creatures live indefinitely? We need to know whether similar genes occur in humans. If so, we would be getting breathtakingly close to reaching the ultimate goal.

We may answer these questions soon, because researchers have found three more genes, *clk-1*, *clk-2*, and *clk-3*, that also control longevity in *Caenorhabditis*. Simultaneous mutation of clk-1 and daf-2 causes nearly a *six-fold rise* in lifespan. In human terms, it would raise life expectancy to 500 years.

Especially exciting is the discovery that human DNA has a gene very similar to the clk-1gene. This is the first step toward finding genes controlling longevity in humans, and it may be a big step toward a life span beyond 300 years. We wouldn't have to damage the genes to bring this about. We could block their action by a drug designed for the purpose. An end to human aging may be close than we can imagine.

In other cells, researchers have found two genes similar to age-1 and daf-2. Deletion of one gene, LAG 1 (longevity assurance gene 1), raises the life span 50 percent. Researchers have made the exciting finding that similar genes occur in several mammals, inlcuding humans. This may be another wedge into the discovery of genes that cause human aging.

These seem to be senescene genes. You damage them, and you live longer, so their function is to limit life. How may they control longevity? Senescense genes may produce suppressors of regulator genes to stop transcription factors. This would shut down cellular genes controlled by the regulator genes, resulting in deterioration and death.

Senescence Gene Produces Suppressor

↓

Regulator Gene Cannot Produce Transcription Factors

↓

Battery of Many Genes Operates Too Slowly To Keep Up with Wear and Tear

↓

Deterioration Of Cells And Death

The way senescence genes operate may be more complex, but their discovery is an exciting step toward the control of human aging. Researchers already know the structure of the LAG 1 gene. It is unlike any gene previously known. Detection of similar genes in animal and human cells tells us this kind of gene is universal, so findings with simple creatures will help to raise human longevity. Probably genes related to age-1, daf-2, and clk-1 limit your life span. Determination of their structures will allow them to be used, along with LAG 1, to discover potential senescence genes in human cells. Research is advancing faster than you may have thought possible toward finding the genes that control human aging.

Longevity Genes And The Lifespan Clock

If genes such as age-1 are truly senescence genes that curtail your life span, then something must keep them from acting until you reach old age. A good possibility is a "longevity gene" that produces a protein to suppress senescence genes. Senescence genes obviously remain switched off until old age. The next question is, what switches them on? What is the clock that controls how long we live? It kills fruit flies after a few weeks, mice after 2 years, and humans after 120 years. We do not know how a cell tells time, but researchers have discovered a possibility. It relates to how many times a cell divides. Human cells in culture divide about fifty times. Toward the end of the series of divisions, they show the same senescence that occurs in aging humans. Cells from increasingly older persons divide fewer times before they die.

How might a limit to cell divisions relate to life span? One way for cells to tell time depends on *telomeres*, DNA segments at the ends of chromosomes. The end of a DNA chain is its Achilles' heel. Damage to the end can wipe out vital genes, but damage usually doesn't occur there because the DNA at the end of a chromosome isn't a gene. Instead, it's a telomere, which isn't a pattern for anything. In humans, it repeats hundreds of times before you get to a gene. Each division of cells causes the destruction of some of the repeating segments in telomeres. Thus, a limit to life comes when the last of a protective telomere is gone and destruction begins on the essential genes near the end of a chromosome. Limiting life by shortening telomeres seems more likely when we see what occurs in cancer cells, which are immortal and divide indefinitely. Cancer cells produce a protein, telomerase, which continually restores the length of telomeres. Evidence that telomeres may be the clock comes from experiments in which researchers lengthened telomeres in old cells. This extended the life of the cells.

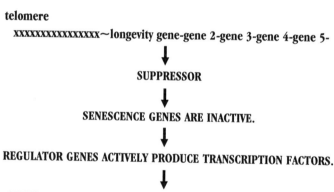

YOUNG CELLS

telomere

xxxxxxxxxxxxxxxx~longevity gene-gene 2-gene 3-gene 4-gene 5-

↓

SUPPRESSOR

↓

SENESCENCE GENES ARE INACTIVE.

↓

REGULATOR GENES ACTIVELY PRODUCE TRANSCRIPTION FACTORS.

↓

GENES ARE FULLY ACTIVE. CELL REPLACES WORN-OUT PROTEINS AND IS PHYSICALLY YOUNG.

Let's combine the findings on genes and longevity to make a simple picture of how genes could limit longevity and cause aging. First, let's examine the activities in young cells.

A longevity gene lies at the end of a chromosome, next to a telomere. It is permanently switched on and produces

OLD CELLS

gene 2-gene 3- gene 4-gene 5

SENESCENCE GENES ARE ACTIVE.
↓
SUPPRESSOR
↓
**REGULATOR GENES ARE INACTIVE,
PRODUCING NO TRANSCRIPTION FACTORS.**

**GENES OPERATE TOO SLOWLY TO REPLACE WEAR AND TEAR.
DEATH ENSUES.**

a suppressor of senescence genes. The suppressor blocks the senescence genes from acting. Regulator genes are free to produce transcription factors. They switch on the cell's genes to produce proteins that constantly replace worn-out proteins. This keeps you physically youthful.

Now, what happens after much time passes? After roughly fifty divisions, the telomere is totally consumed, and the longevity gene adjacent to it is destroyed. The longevity gene no longer produces a suppressor to stop the senescence genes.

No longer blocked by a suppressor from the longevity gene, the senescence gene is now free to produce its own suppressor. This suppressor stops the production of transcription factors by regulator genes. Without transcription factors, the cell's genes produce so few new proteins that they can't replace worn-out ones. The cell's proteins degrade, resulting in deterioration and death.

The real picture is certainly more complex, but in science you begin with the simplest explanation. As we discover more, the picture will become clear.

Life Extension By Controlling Gene Expression

As we find out more about how genes regulate longevity, our prospects of controlling aging will continually brighten. There are many ways we could do it. I will list three, but there are a zillion clever people in the world, and they are certain to come up with many more.

One approach is to find substances that switch on cellular genes, prevent the suppression of regulatory genes, or switch off senescence genes. One place such substances may occur is in young cells. Researchers have sought these substances by extracting the nuclei of young cells and testing whether the extracts would switch genes from old cells back on. The young cell extract restored about a third of gene activity. This is far from the level of young cells, but it is a start. If purified, the factor might be more effective. Other factors may be better. For example, researchers have reported that centrophenoxine restores mRNA formation in old rats to the level in young ones. In preparations of genes from old cells, other researchers have found centrophenoxine also returns mRNA synthesis to its level in young cells. This may be why centrophenoxine extends the life of laboratory animals. Thus, we might switch genes back on after aging switches them off. If so, there are probably substances far more effective and stable than centrophenoxine. This raises the prospect of a drug that can slow aging.

A better approach may be to block the action of senescence genes. Certain kinds of old cells contain high levels of mRNA for a protein that is a potent inhibitor of cell division. In contrast, cells transformed to the cancerous (immortal) state contain no mRNA for this protein. Researchers have made an *antisense DNA* for the mRNA for this protein. Antisense DNA binds to and ties up a specific mRNA, in this case an mRNA for the protein. When they treated old cells with the antisense DNA, it stopped senescence and caused the cells to multiply again. Instead of appearing old, they looked young. The treatment didn't transform cells to cancer. The removal of antisense DNA changed them back to an aged state. *Antisense DNA dou-*

bled the life span of the human cells. More treatment with antisense DNA might have extended the lifespan further. This is an important finding, not because antisense DNA for this mRNA will extend life but because it shows a way to control senescence genes by binding the mRNA they produce. First, we must identify senescence genes (like the human equivalent of age-1) whose mRNAs must be tied up. Second, we must be able to deliver antisense DNAs into our cells. Then, regular treatment with antisense DNAs could extend life indefinitely.

Finally, we could insert longevity genes into cells under independent control. The first two means to halt aging employ a drug or antisense DNA. These methods would require you to take a capsule or an injection regularly. The ideal situation is to halt aging permanently. Researchers have already advanced toward this goal. One group has taken genes for an elongation protein (which helps ribosomes make proteins) and has altered their control regions so that they are permanently switched on. Inserted into fruit flies, they slowed aging and caused the maximum lifespan to rise 42 percent. If the same technique worked in health-conscious humans, it could raise life expectancy to nearly 150 years and the maximum life span to 170 years. Another group has inserted into fruit flies additional copies of genes for proteins that protect against oxidation. The maximum life span rose 34 percent.

These effects came from the insertion of cellular genes. What might happen if we were to insert longevity genes? In the scheme outlined above, insertion of longevity genes into protected areas of chromosomes could, barring disease or an accident, extend life indefinitely. At the rate gene therapy is advancing, this should be possible by the time we identify the genes that cause aging.

The Road Ahead

To get a sense of what is ahead, we should look back

at how fast we have progressed. In 1975 we had growing evidence that genes control longevity, but we had no idea what genes are involved. We were occupied with discovering how aging changes activities inside cells. By 1985, researchers were identifying genes whose expression fell in old age. Most retained 10-50 percent of their activity, indicating the fall in expression resulted from the loss of a transcription factor. By 1995, the number of genes known to switch off partially had grown rapidly. Researchers had found that senescent cells switch off several of their regulator genes that each control large groups of genes. Of enormous importance was the discovery of genes that control longevity. Age-1, daf-2, and LAG 1 are genes in simple organisms. But the finding of similar genes in mammalian and human cells indicates that age-1, daf-2, and clk-1 will lead us to the genes controlling human longevity. Considering that the control of genes that govern longevity will eliminate aging, the advances between 1985 and 1995 were immense.

All evidence points to even greater advances in coming years. We should identify the genes that control longevity in simple organisms. We should use not only LAG 1, but also age-1, daf-2, and similar genes to find out whether they have counterparts in mammals and humans. We should know whether these genes cause senescence by producing suppressors of regulator genes or whether they act in some other way. We may also know whether there is a longevity gene that keeps senescence genes suppressed until old age and how telomere length, or another mechanism, controls it.

Beyond 2005, as we learn still more about the genes that cause aging, the search will likely be for ways to control aging and extend longevity for many years. Although centrophenoxine is an unlikely candidate, we may find other drugs that block the action of senescence genes. These might include antisense DNA, but the problem of getting intact DNA into all cells of the body is formidable. But the discovery of substances that stop the action of senescence genes may lead to blocking drugs, a daily dose of which extends youthful life for decades. After the next decade, we should isolate longevity genes that suppress senescence genes in early life. We should progress on the difficult task of inserting them, permanently switched on, into all cells to replace the longevity genes switched off by aging. This is a huge problem, and it may take decades to solve. But later in the twenty-first century, we should control aging by gene therapy. Within a decade after that, a permanent halt to senescence using gene therapy should be widely available. This will extend life indefinitely.

Will this be immortality? The dictionary defines *immortality* as "endless life or existence." Cessation of aging will not halt deaths from diseases or accidents. It may be possible in the future to eliminate deaths from diseases, but even the most optimistic projections don't envision an end to accidental deaths. Still, people will likely average more than 300 years, possibly as many as 500 years. The reward of research on senescence genes is enormous, but we have further to go than for any other way to extend life. Better approaches will appear. They won't occur overnight. But, considering how fast we have moved recently, strong efforts could yield rapid progress in the next 20 years. It won't be immortality, but it will be as close to immortality as you can get.

11

Changing The Course Of History

*The major advances in civilization are processes that all
but wreck the societies in which they occur.*
—Alfred North Whitehead, *Adventures in Ideas*

At its climax, the rise in longevity that has now begun will
have the greatest impact of any event in history. Governments already are struggling to cope with the growing mass
of people living past 65. They are just beginning to feel the
impact of the dramatic rise in persons living beyond 85. But
these are only the first stirrings of a vast cataclysm. Spectacular progress in medicine is heading toward the conquest of
most diseases in the foreseeable future. Advances against
aging are heading us toward a world of physically young
persons, their lives limited only by accidents or unexpected
diseases. These events will affect every aspect of social, economic, and personal life. They will first shatter, then transform, society.

The Rise In Longevity

The advance toward life without limit will occur in two
phases. The phases will overlap, but they will have vastly
different effects on you. In the first phase, longevity will

rise with the rise in the conquest of diseases. It has been underway for 300 years, but in the past 50 years it has skyrocketed. Newspapers and television report daily on major advances against a variety of diseases. The result of all the progress is the ability to live progressively further past 100. Unless financial support of medical research halts (an unlikely possibility), we will see the conquest of diseases extending life to 120-130. Although people living past 100 can be healthy and active, the aging process will cause them to become increasingly frail as they pass 100 and approach 120. A growing population of 100 to 120-year-olds, even a growing population over 65, is already having an impact. But the imminent social and economic impacts will be huge—some positive, many negative. Thus, it is essential that we move into the second phase as quickly as possible.

In the second phase, the rise in longevity will come from the ever greater control of aging. It will probably begin around 2030, although unexpected advances could bring it earlier. At that point, your life expectancy will climb rapidly from the growing conquest of aging and diseases. Over the following 50 years, the combination will extend life to 300 and beyond. Its impact on society, the economy, and your life will be immense, shattering, and mostly positive. Let's look at some effects of the two phases.

Effects Of Longevity On Population

The usual reaction to the thought of people living far longer is that it will cause a population explosion. But compared with the current eruption of the world's population, it will have only a modest impact from now until well past 2050. It took humans thousands of years to reach 1 billion people in 1800, but only 130 years to attain 2 billion in 1930. We achieved 3 billion by 1960, 4 billion by 1975, and 5 billion by 1987. Only a small part of this immense rise came during a time when medicine advanced rapidly and had the greatest effect on extending life. Instead, it is the result of unrestrained reproduction. As the alien from space says, "They began with 2 people, and now they have 5 billion. Someone should have turned the hose on them."

In the United States, with a population of 249 million in 1990, one estimate projects the complete elimination of the five leading causes of death (which would raise life expectancy to 100) would add 7 million over a 25-year period. At the same time, net immigration (legal and illegal) would add 23 million. So, extending life will have a relatively small effect until we control aging. Even then, modulating factors such as accidents, homicides, and unexpected diseases will minimize the contribution of longevity to population growth until sometime beyond 2050.

Eventually, when aging is under control, stringent restriction on births will be necessary. Otherwise, the human population will expand to a point that exceeds the earth's capacity. Of course, we could with difficulty colonize the moon and Mars. But birth control is more likely by personal choice. Few people who have already raised a family would look forward with enthusiasm to hundreds of years spent raising more children. The world is far too attractive, and they would already have their original family. Far more urgent is the need for nations today to exercise even modest control of reproduction. The problem of population growth is unrestrained procreation, not life extension.

Effects Of Longevity On The Economy

If the effects of life extension on an already burgeoning population are relatively small, its potential effects on the economy are large. Even the first phase could bankrupt Social Security and retirement annuity funds unless the government and the insurance industry act to prevent it.

Employment

Life extension will have one of its greatest effects on the outlook for jobs. Recall that a shutdown of the genes that cause aging will make your body's cells the same as those of a young person. You will be physically young regardless of your age. Many people today enjoy their jobs. When they retire, they often feel lost, even devastated. Faced with the "youthful" ability to work, many may opt to continue working for personal satisfaction and a sense of belonging. The fact that they are youthful and possess decades of skill, experience, and judgment will also make them attractive to employers.

The net effect will likely be for people to remain in the workforce much longer. This could reduce the opportunities for young persons entering the workforce. Unemployment could soar to levels above those of the Great Depression. To give young people opportunities, it may be necessary to restrict immigration severely to keep immigrants from competing for the diminishing pool of jobs. An enormous effort by the government will probably be necessary to create new jobs through economic expansion. In an emergency, something similar to the Works Progress Administration of the 1930s (which was far more successful than often supposed) may be necessary for a time. President Bill Clinton's proposals for innovations to produce new industries for the global market could also ease the employment crunch. In addition, some workers may accumulate enough annuities to retire and live on dividends, even if their life expectancy is 300.

Retirement

Life extension will have an equally-great effect on retirement. Social Security is the first thing that comes to mind when you think of retirement in the United States. The intent of the Social Security Act of 1935 was to establish a retirement program for American workers. But by

1985 it was providing retirement benefits to workers and survivors, disability insurance, health insurance, supplemental funds for lower-income persons, unemployment compensation, aid to lower-income families with dependent children, free medical care for welfare recipients, social services, maternal and child health, and services for crippled children. To cover this, the Social Security tax rose from 1 percent of your salary in 1937 to 7.65 percent in 1990. About 124 million people contribute. Thirty-seven million, only a part retirees, get cash benefits.

Before we even consider the problems brought on by increased longevity, we can see that Social Security is threatened today by problems from the growing number of people who receive benefits (especially welfare benefits) but have contributed nothing to the program. This is due partly to the influx of unskilled immigrants, legal and illegal, who cannot find work in a job market shrinking from downsizing and robots. It is also due to citizens unemployed for the same reasons. It is further due to the expanded eligibility for disability payments to include, for example, drug addiction, chronic fatigue syndrome, and obesity.

On top of these problems, we have those resulting from rising life expectancy. In 1935, when Social Security began, life expectancy was 62 years. Starting retirement payments at 65 made it probable that the payments would not last long. But now life expectancy is 76, and for health-conscious people is 100. Retirement payments already last far longer than originally assumed.

These happenings are massive threats to Social Security. To save the program, the U.S. Congress has curtailed benefits, taxed some benefits, and put in motion a gradual increase in the retirement age from 65 to 67. This will not be enough. The only thing that has saved Social Security has been the failure of most people to be health-conscious. If even half the population began living to 100, Social

Security could not keep up. As longevity of 100-120 years becomes common, the elimination of disability payments for the physically fit, the elimination of early retirement at 62, and a rising retirement age to 70 or higher will be required. This should keep the program solvent until approximately 2050.

Annuities and other private plans for retirement will have equal financial pressures during the first phase, but they will cope far better. They will not have to pay out to welfare programs. They will have the flexible management to respond as life expectancy rises. Still, their response will require either higher premiums for retirement at 65 or the postponement of retirement until age 70 or beyond. It is likely that postponement will rise steadily above the age of 70. We will likely see retirement ages rise to 85, 100, and even 150 during the early stages of the control of aging.

The second phase of life extension will force a revolution in retirement. If we are lucky, the increasing control of aging will extend life in phases, perhaps to 150, then to 180, then to 300 and beyond. Still, we will probably have to face an indefinite lifespan sometime in the last half of the twenty-first century. Funded retirement at age 65 will long since have become infeasible because people could not pay premiums high enough for an indefinite lifespan. People will opt to retire later.

Insurance

Life extension will also have an enormous effect on the huge insurance industry. It will involve millions of people and enormous amounts of investment capital.

Life insurance companies, through no fault of their own, will reap a bonanza of premiums and profits from increased longevity. Why? Life insurance premiums are calculated from mortality tables, which show the number of people in each age and gender group that die each year. An actuary, a person trained to make life expectancy calculations, estimates the number of premiums the insurance company must collect annually from each group. Actuaries ensure the premiums and their earned interest not only equal the benefits to be paid to the policyholders' beneficiaries but also cover company expenses and contingencies. Life expectancy tables tend to lag several years behind mortality because of the time required to collect accurate mortality data and to calculate probabilities. If life expectancy rises rapidly, premiums will still be based on dated mortality tables, resulting in higher premiums than needed. But it will not take the industry long to focus on a 100 to 120-year life expectancy, which should result in much lower premiums than today.

A revolution in life insurance will come during the second phase of life extension. An increase in life expectancy to 180 or more years will probably cause all life insurance policies to become limited payment policies. These will be paid up after premium payments for a certain number of years (often 20) unless the insured person dies sooner. If you are expected to live 300 years, the interest on twenty years of extremely low premiums will easily cover the insurance benefit This is likely to make life insurance almost universal, inexpensive, and greatly expand investment capital.

Health insurance costs should continue to rise in the near future due to the rising costs of treating smokers and others who are not health conscious. Costs may also rise because mounting numbers of persons over age 65 mean surging numbers who need long-term care for stroke, arthritis, Alzheimer's, or other disabling diseases.

The cost of health insurance will hinge on how many people are health conscious. The more people who don't smoke, avoid secondary smoke, exercise, maintain ideal weight, have a medical exam annually, immunize against diseases, and follow the advice of their physicians, the lower will be health insurance premiums. Being health conscious reduces the huge costs of health care. If we must treat diseases instead of preventing them, costs soar. In the United States, it costs $95 million to treat cardiovascular disease, but 80 percent is preventable. It costs $100 million to treat cancer, but 70 percent is preventable. It costs $26 million to treat AIDS, but 99 percent is preventable. In fact, Dr. C. Everett Koop, former Surgeon General of the United States, and a group of medical experts say that 70 percent of all illness is preventable. Yearly medical costs for a health-conscious person average $190, while those for a person with unhealthy habits average $1,550. Anything that prevents a disease saves enormous amounts of your money. It costs a pharmaceutical company an average of $231 million to develop a new drug, but if it prevents expensive treatment, it cuts your health care costs. Thus, we must prevent diseases and develop less expensive treatments (drugs instead of surgery, for example). But the most important way to save money on health care is a healthy lifestyle.

Still, to take advantage of the growing ability to extend life, you must have access to good health care. As of 1996, almost every developed nation has systems to accomplish this. The United States, despite having some of the best medical talent and facilities in the world, has a failed system. It depends on insurance companies whose goal is maximum profit. Many charge high premiums, avoid paying benefits, and seek to insure only healthy people. Administrative costs averaged 20 percent of the total cost, while the administrative cost of the government's Medicare program is only 7 percent. Premiums in the United States have risen so high that nearly 40 million people cannot afford health insurance. Hospitals and physicians have to shift the cost of treating uninsured people to the insured, raising premiums higher. This has forced more people to drop their insurance. The cost of health care has risen toward a trillion dollars.

The situation has evoked many solutions. Some have urged the adoption of the Canadian tax-supported plan. But conservative congressmen have screamed, "Socialized medicine!" (By the way, both Congress and the military have socialized medicine.) Health maintenance organizations (HMOs) have claimed lower premiums, but physicians complain that HMOs have done it by curbing treatment. Curtailing treatment to save money is a step downward for the nation that sees itself as the world's leader. Some conservatives have even proposed to limit health care for old adults since, it is argued, they will die anyway. This is a giant step down a slope toward gas chambers and ovens. It drew a sharp reply in the *New England Journal of Medicine:*

> In some primitive societies, the elderly acquiesced in the limitation of their lifespans by abandonment. The ethos of death as a communal act may have been an appropriate response to extreme scarcity in certain, primitive societies. The wealthiest country in history should not go back to that future.

In 1993 President Clinton, with the advice of hundreds of experts in finance and medicine, proposed a system of insurance-purchasing alliances that would have left the health care system intact at a lower cost. Faced with the loss of profits, the insurance industry spent millions on television attack ads. Instead of fixing the plan's faults, Republican congressmen killed it for political gain. As a result, more people lost their health insurance. Costs soared. It was a shameful chapter in American history.

A civilized nation has good health care for everyone. There are many excellent systems to provide it. Until it occurs, Americans' potential for longevity will not be attained.

As diseases are overcome, health care costs will begin to fall. The elimination of most cardiovascular disease will save $95 million of America's $700 million health care costs. The conquest of cancer will save $100 million, and the conquest of other diseases will reduce costs further. Continued progress in medicine will then cause a long decline in health care costs to surprisingly low levels. As this occurs, health insurance providers will prosper as never before, despite decreasing premiums for Medicare and health insurance, because it will cost them so little to provide health care. We already see this when a drug cures a disease and prevents major surgery. As we control diseases and aging, health care costs for astonishingly good care will plummet.

Commerce

Those few economists who have looked at the startling possibility of living longer foresee it to have an overall positive effect on the economy. Initially, its effects will be unfavorable in some areas but then will become steadily better. In the near future, businesses that cater to the elderly (retirement and nursing homes, assisted care, medicine, hospitals, and tour operators) will flourish. But as we overcome diseases and begin to slow aging, many of those will decline. Businesses that cater to more active persons (automobiles, entertainment, sports) will grow.

As people live longer, they will be continuing consumers of all manner of merchandise. Pictures of seniors today eking along on Social Security are not the norm. Most have other income. Seniors are the top market for goods and services. Their steady demand for merchandise will be joined by younger persons becoming buyers to produce an overall growth in commerce. This growth in commerce will extend to the massive housing industry. As longevity rises, people will occupy their residences years longer instead of putting them up for sale. Younger persons will also be a larger market for newly built housing, stimulating the construction industry and the vast set of businesses that supply it.

Rising longevity will also stimulate transportation, whether the elderly travel while still employed or join the growing number of retirees who use cruise ships, aircraft, rail, motor homes, automobiles, and guided tours. Older persons tend to be enthusiastic travelers. They also tend to be enthusiastic vacationers, using the income from a lifetime of investment. This will stimulate the leisure industry as well. Education should expand as older persons return to school for career changes. Publishing, art, and theater should likewise prosper from the quest of older persons for knowledge and entertainment.

Another positive aspect for the economy is that older persons are usually careful financial managers and investors. This will provide more investment capital for development. Economists say it will increase the communication and transportation systems that aid the exchange of ideas. This will add to our store of knowledge, stimulating scientific and technological progress, which hikes productivity.

Finally, older persons with substantial experience in a field will be likely innovators of new products and businesses. The lifelong experience of older workers and their tendency to innovate has been called by economist Julian Simon the "ultimate resource." This may be one of the saving features for employment of younger persons in new industries that result from innovation. Overall, the more we extend life by blocking aging, the better the effect on the economy.

Effect Of Longevity On Society

The extension of life will have an enormous effect on relationships among people. In the first phase, as the population of obviously elderly people grows, increasing conflict is likely. We see the beginnings today in the resentment toward the retired elderly living the good life in Florida by younger people who contribute to Social Security and fear it won't be there when they retire. Ageism is a hurtful, discriminatory attitude. On television and elsewhere the elderly are portrayed as obstinate, bumbling idiots. It has been described expertly by Dr. Robert Butler, former Director of the National Institute on Aging, in his Pulitzer Prize-winning book *Why Survive? Being Old in America*. But the elderly are striking back through political action. The high percentage of elderly people who vote gives them political power beyond their numbers. As their numbers increase, this power should increase, causing more conflict.

Once we control aging, attitudes based on appearance will disappear since the unthinkable will have occurred. The appearance and activity of a 150-year-old will match those of a 25-year-old. The resentment toward retired people should decrease because even a 150-year life expectancy will rule out retirement at 65.

Still, barring a miracle, economic conflict over jobs will probably boil over into bitter social conflict between the experienced, physically young elderly and youths who make their usual rebellion against society's customs. Imagine a 150-year-old in 2100 insisting on music by the Beatles.

The control of aging may also lead to interesting associations of 180-year-old, physically young women with 30-year-old men, or 180-year-old physically young men with 30-year-old women. For married couples, more decades together, possibly dozens more, may strain some marriages but strengthen others.

Effect Of Longevity On Your Personal Life

Imagine how you would feel if you were the physical equal of a 20-year-old, and knew you would remain that way. Think of a typical day for you in 2050. Longer life will give you the opportunity to go more places, meet more people, have more experiences, read more books, listen to more music, enjoy more art, have more romance, and do myriad other things. The door will be open for more education, probably in fields you had always wanted to try.

There will be the opportunity for new careers, perhaps several careers in a lifetime, or for multiple changes in lifestyle. Some, of course, may regard longer life as more years of boredom and choose not to take action to live longer. That should be an option. But most people will take the first opportunity in history to do everything they ever have wanted to do. All it will take is time, and you will have plenty of it.

Assessing The Impact Of The Rise In Longevity

Unfortunately, neither government nor anyone else has done much to determine the impact of today's rising longevity. Planning for the even greater impact of controlling aging has fared even worse.

Few people have seriously considered the possibility that an extension of life will occur. Even among gerontologists, more attention is paid to the social and psychological problems of the elderly than to controlling the aging that causes those problems. A former head of the National Institute on Aging was fond of saying its mission was to "add life to years, not years to life." One elderly gerontologist has stated that he can't understand why we would want to control aging.

Yet our ability to extend life will roll forward like a juggernaut. We must prepare for it, lest it overwhelms our economic, political, and social institutions. In his book *Maximum Life Span*, Dr. Roy Walford, a brilliant gerontologist at UCLA, relates how he was the only biologist appointed to a National Academy of Science Committee on Aging, whose task was to advise the U.S. Government. Despite hard arguing, he failed to convince the other committee members that they should discuss the impact of the extension of life. They couldn't imagine it happening.

Measures that could help cope with the rise in longevity have so far fared poorly. Universal health insurance could not only save enormous amounts of money but also could provide a mechanism to react to rapid advances in life extension. But universal health care in the United States was torpedoed in 1993. Nearly all developed nations have it. Americans will now likely suffer the most. But in all nations, many physicians assume life expectancy will be only 75-80 years. So they stop the aggressive treatment of patients over 65 because they believe these patients will soon die anyway.

In view of the massive impact of longer life, we need to study the consequences of rising longevity. We need to do it soon. Hear the rumble of far-off thunder on a hot July night, after the weather bureau has warned of severe storms. We may choose to deny or ignore the threat. But the sudden roar of a tornado will tell us it's too late to prepare.

12

The Future

In a time of exploding change—with personal lives being torn apart, the existing social order crumbling, and a fantastic new way of life emerging on the horizon—asking the very largest of questions about our future is not merely a matter of intellectual curiosity. It is a matter of survival.
—Alvin Toffler, *The Third Wave*

We must look toward the future. Each passing hour takes us there. What lies ahead is a question as important as any we can ask. But when we look forward, we must be careful to go no further than an extension of the facts permits. At the same time, we must guard against the closed mind syndrome, a refusal to accept that advances at the present rate will probably continue. We must also keep in mind that a population does not have a uniform life expectancy (76 years, for example). It's a spectrum, from 100 for health-conscious people to no better than 50 for obese, sedentary smokers.

The following projections apply to health-conscious nonsmokers. How far can we extend their lives in 2010 or 2030 by continued progress against diseases? How far can we extend life in 2030 or 2050 by advances against aging?

Since research on both proceeds concurrently, what is their combined effect?

These are not idle questions. Watch the advances in medicine reported in your newspaper for a month. Then remember that you have seen only a tiny fraction of what is happening in thousands of laboratories around the world. It is only when you have read the torrent of new findings in hundreds of biomedical journals every week and daily on the Internet that you realize how fast we are moving. Of course, we can't predict the future with certainty. When we project the future, we move from fact to theory. Still, theories are an essential part of science. Projections based on today's trends are the best pictures we have of the future. Nothing is guaranteed, but we can see a likely future for health-conscious people. Progress may be faster than projected. It often is. It also may be slower if we run into unexpected obstacles. With this in mind, let's look ahead.

Life Extension In 2000

Historians will look back on 2000 as the time when the longevity of health-conscious people began an ever faster rise due to the conquest of diseases and aging. Figure 12-1 shows the starting points for the future conquest of diseases. The starting points are not the barriers faced by the general population (dark bars). They are the barriers faced by the health-conscious population (light bars) because we already can prevent or cure 80 percent of cardiovascular disease, 60 percent of cancer, 70 percent of stroke, 65 percent of accidents, 90 percent of chronic lung disease, 90 percent of pneumonia, 85 percent of diabetes, 99 percent of AIDS, 70 percent of suicide, and 80 percent of chronic liver disease. It is a brighter picture than we might expect for the beginning of the twenty-first century.

Aging likely kills a significant fraction of the health-conscious population over age 80. Medicine won't prevent it in

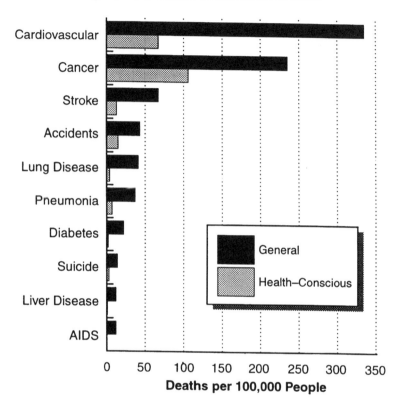

Figure 12-1. Status of Diseases in 2000

2000, but research is progressing against it. We have already extended the lives of laboratory animals (in some cases doubling their life spans) by dietary restriction or with the drugs deprenyl, centrophenoxine, and ethoxyquin. We step into the twenty-first century knowing much about what occurs in aging cells. We have found two, and possibly three, causes of aging: oxidation, the failure of protein synthesis, and possibly the failure of DNA repair. We have traced the failures to switched-off genes, and we have found genes that may cause aging when triggered by a cellular clock. An antisense DNA to one gene has doubled the life span of human cells, while action on senescence genes has quadrupled the life of a simple creature. We even have found hints of the final piece in the puzzle, the longevity clock. Drugs to slow human aging will not be practicable in 2000. But the reward to the pharmaceutical company that finds one will be billions of dollars since most everyone wants to live longer. Will an antioxidant or deprenyl be the first to slow human aging? Will a combination?

Recall that for health-conscious people in 2000,

- Life expectancy at birth is 100.

- A 35-year-old can expect to live to 101.

- A 65-year-old can expect to live to 104.

The maximum lifespan may not rise above 120, although someone born in 1875 might reach 125. Still, a health-conscious 35-year-old in 2000 can expect to live until 2066, when the outlook for long life should be very bright. With drugs that slow aging in laboratory animals and genes that control longevity, we head into the twenty-first century toward the conquest of aging.

Life Extension In 2030

Many of you reading this will be alive in 2030. By then, medicine's golden age will have advanced 30 years beyond its level in 2000. Its gains will have a major effect on diseases. Also, 30 years of research may see the first drugs to slow human aging. For longevity, the era from 2000 to 2030 will likely be the dawn of the most eventful changes in history.

Prevention And Cure Of Diseases

From the threshold of medicine in 2000, 30 years' progress in prevention and treatment projects far fewer deaths from diseases. Organ transplants will be routine. Electromechanical organs and body parts will be reliable and widely used. We will grow new organs for you in the laboratory, heading toward the regular replacement of injured, defective, or diseased organs of all sorts. Gene therapy, in its infancy in 2000, should cure dozens of diseases. The structure of human DNA—every gene—will be known. Each protein in your cells will have been cataloged. With this knowledge, we will fully understand life and diseases. Medicine will change. It will start to treat the body as a complex machine that benefits from routine test and repair, directed and analyzed by computers.

Cardiovascular Disease

Our ability to prevent or cure cardiovascular disease climbed from 60 percent in 1980 to 70 percent in 1990 and will rise to 80 percent in 2000. All evidence suggests this trend will continue, although at a somewhat slower pace. New cholesterol-lowering drugs will prevent atherosclerosis, clean out atherosclerotic deposits in your blood vessels, and wipe out atherosclerosis. Other new drugs will stop hypertension. Cardiologists will cure heart attacks with speedy clot busters and angioplasty. Growth factor therapy after a heart attack will repair all damage. Personal kits will monitor your heart condition and will provide drugs and equipment to keep your heart going during a suspected attack until you can reach a hospital. Heart failure and other cardiac disorders will be the targets of much research between 2000 and 2030. New heart valves will prevent many cases of heart failure. Growth factors and drugs will stop cardiomyopathy, while drugs increasingly will control arrhythmia.

Figure 12-2 extends the past rate of decline in cardiovascular deaths down to 30 percent of the 1980 rate by 2010, to 15 percent by 2020, and to 10 percent by 2030. Dr. Jeffrey Fisher in *Rx 2000* goes further. After consulting many medical researchers, he predicts we will wipe out 99 percent of deaths from cardiovascular disease by 2030.

Figure 12-2. Projected Drop in Major Diseases

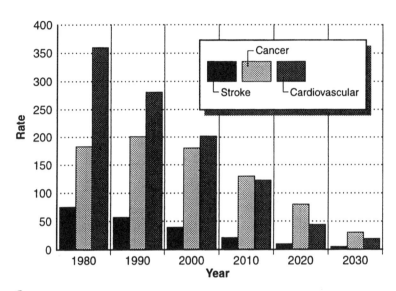

Cancer

The trend shows our ability to prevent or treat cancer has climbed from 45 percent in 1980, to 50 percent in 1990 and will rise to 60 percent in 2000. During the 1990s, laboratories have produced a flood of promising treatments based on molecular biology. After 2000, two factors will govern how rapidly we conquer cancer. First, how fast will we find the cause and means to prevent each type of cancer? Second, how rapidly will new treatments (specific antibodies, tumor suppressor genes, antisense DNA, altered viruses, and anticancer drugs) come into widespread use? By 2030, we should know the causes of almost all cancers, and we will have 30 years of improved prevention. Cancer cures should be routine, as specific antibodies, gene therapy, antisense DNA, and drugs will be in full use and soon surpassed by newer methods.

Figure 12-2 shows the trend of cancer deaths falling to

35 percent of their 1980 rate by 2010 and to 15 percent by 2030. With the advice of many researchers, Dr. Fisher in *Rx 2000* predicts 75 percent of cancer deaths will be gone by 2010 and 99 percent by 2030.

Stroke

Figure 12-2 shows that deaths from stroke had dropped 24 percent by 1990 and have continued to fall. The ability to prevent strokes has climbed from 50 percent in 1980 to 80 percent today. This trend should continue as we reduce atherosclerosis and hypertension. By 2010, stroke should be 30 percent of its 1980 level and should be a rare disease by 2030. For strokes that do occur, drugs will repair the damage.

Thus, three diseases that cause 64 percent of deaths should almost be gone by 2030. This is similar to the drop in the leading killers of 1900 (pneumonia, tuberculosis, and typhus) between 1900 and 1940.

Chronic Lung Disease

We can prevent 90 percent of chronic lung disease today. More control of secondary smoke and air pollution and progress toward cures for chronic bronchitis, asthma, and emphysema could essentially eliminate deaths by 2030.

Accidents

We can now prevent 65 percent of the accidental deaths of 1920. Progress with safer vehicles, the prevention of drunk driving, electronic controls on highways, high-speed rail, and safety in the home and factory should reduce accidental deaths in 2030 by 50 percent. The decline of cardiovascular disease, cancer, and stroke may leave accidents as the leading cause of death.

Pneumonia

Our ability to prevent or cure pneumonia has risen from 50 percent in 1980 to 80 percent today. Further improvement of vaccines should prevent almost all pneumonia and influenza by 2030. Newer antibiotics, plus vitamins and drugs to keep immunity high, will cure pneumonia we do not prevent.

Diabetes

There has been a decline among health-conscious people in the 93 percent of diabetes that is not-insulin-dependent (type II), but no decrease in insulin-dependent diabetes (type I). By 2010, pancreatic cell implants may abolish the need for insulin injections and control type I diabetes. By 2030, gene therapy should control type I.

AIDS

By 2030, prevention will still be the most effective way to abolish AIDS. Research on the disease should produce a vaccine to wipe out deaths.

Suicide

Beginning with our ability to prevent 70 percent of suicides, continued advances in the detection and treatment of depression should reduce suicide deaths steadily. By 2030, unless unexpected stresses hit us, suicides should be less than 50 percent of their current rate.

Chronic Liver Disease

Beginning with our ability to prevent 80 percent of liver disease, continued efforts to lower heavy drinking, to prevent hepatitis, and to develop growth factors to restore damaged livers, will eliminate almost all chronic liver disease.

In 2030 the ten leading causes of death in the 1990s, responsible for 81 percent of all deaths, should be mostly gone. Research will have advanced against dozens of other diseases that each cause less than 1 percent of all deaths but together cause the other 19 percent. Continuation of current progress should wipe out 50 percent of infectious diseases and cure 25 percent of other diseases, including septicemia, Alzheimer's disease, cystic fibrosis, multiple sclerosis, muscular dystrophy, arthritis, and osteoporosis. Gene therapy should erase most inherited diseases and should move fast to delete the rest. We face the prospect of a steep decline in deaths from diseases by 2030.

Prevention of Aging In 2030

While we progress against diseases, researchers will continue to progress against aging. By 2030, we should understand the aging process and its control. We should know the genes involved and be able to control them in the laboratory.

The first anti-aging drugs to pass the long testing process for approval by the U.S. Food and Drug Administration may be antioxidants or deprenyl-like drugs. An antioxidant may raise the life expectancy of health-conscious 35-year-olds to 135. Improving on vitamin E and thymosin, new drugs may keep the immune system from declining. We should be well along on the development of other drugs to slow aging, and one or more may be in use. Anti-aging drugs will raise the life expectancy from the conquest of diseases in 2030 beyond the 114 years for a health-conscious 35-year-old. For example, a follow-up to deprenyl designed to slow aging may boost the longevity of health-conscious 35-year-olds to around 150.

More effective may be substances that block a gene that causes senescence. Even if partly effective, they should extend life astonishingly. Since we have found genes linked to senescence in the 1990s, it is likely that 35 years later, in 2030, research to block senescence genes will be very active. It should have found drugs that block the genes in laboratory animals. These may extend the lives of animals remarkably, but they will probably not yet be ready for human use.

Life Expectancy In 2030

By 2030, we should have overcome diseases and slowed aging to produce an impressive rise in longevity.

From progress since 2000 against diseases, health-conscious persons who use the methods of 2030 for prevention and cure can extend life further past 100.

- Life expectancy at birth will be 103 years.
- A 35-year-old can expect to live to 114.
- An 85-year-old can expect to live to 117.

Someone born in 1900 might reach a maximum lifespan of 130. For persons using all of the means of 2030 to prevent and cure diseases, the advent of anti-aging drugs should raise longevity 20 percent more.

- Life expectancy at birth will be 130 years.
- A 35-year-old can expect to live to 137.
- An 85-year-old can expect to live to 140.

Although continued progress against diseases will occur, the ability to slow the aging process will be a giant force for extending life. It will change the course of history as humans make the first step toward the long life we have desired for centuries. Since anti-aging drugs extend the youthful phase of life, they will have enormous effects on society.

Life Extension In 2050

Twenty years have passed since 2030. Medicine has changed so much that a physician of the 1990s would have difficulty recognizing it. Twenty years of advances beyond 2030 (50 years beyond 2000) should result in drugs and technology able to prevent and cure most diseases. Prevention will be aided by home monitors that measure dozens of your vital activities and detect abnormalities early enough for treatment before a disease becomes serious. You will transmit the output of these monitors to a computer in your physician's office. The computer will analyze the findings and alert you and your physician to any hint of impending trouble.

Medical knowledge will be so huge that a physician will

be unable to grasp the vast information in a specialty. For a time, from 2000 to 2030, medical specialties may divide rapidly to try to keep up. But by 2050, only the memory and analytical powers of a computer will comprehend medical knowledge. Physicians will use computers and computer networks to aid them in diagnosis and treatment. As medicine uses the vast memory of computers for diagnosis and treatment, physicians will spend more time as internists or family practitioners. Impersonal treatment should give way to caring treatment. As John Naisbitt has predicted in *Megatrends*, the advent of high-tech medicine will lead to "high-touch" attention by physicians.

By 2050, deaths from the leading killers of 2000 and 50 percent of all other diseases should be rare. For each person, the computer-supervised prevention and cure of diseases should resemble the tender, caring maintenance of a complex machine.

By 2050 life extenders, follow-ups to antioxidants and deprenyl, may have been in use for decades to push life expectancy at birth past 130 years. But the big boosts in life will result from blocking the genes that cause aging. Fifty years of progress beyond 2000 will clarify how genes control longevity. Research will find drugs that stop aging in laboratory animals by blocking the genes that cause aging. By 2050, some will be in use. For example, if there is a human analogue of the age-1 gene, a drug that blocks its action might raise life expectancy to 170 years. If there is a human counterpart of the *daf-2/daf-12* combination, stopping their action may push life expectancy to 500 years.

Twenty years of progress in research beyond 2030, high-tech medicine, and few deaths from diseases will extend healthy life remarkably. Accidents, murders, and aging will still kill us, but disease will kill fewer people. Although only 50 years have passed, people will look back on 2000 as we today regard the 1890s. For health-conscious people, the ability to prevent or cure 50 percent of all diseases will contribute to a further rise in life expectancy. From the conquest of diseases alone,

- Life expectancy at birth will be 107 years.
- A 35-year-old can expect to live to 125.
- An 85-year-old can expect to live to 129.
- Someone born in 1910 may reach a maximum life span of 140.

But life expectancy will get a boost from drugs to control the genes that cause aging. Figure 12-3 shows the possible effects of drugs on the longevity of health-conscious people. They will begin with a life expectancy at birth of 107 years. An antioxidant or other drug to diminish the effects of aging should raise the life expectancy of health-conscious people to around 130 years. A 35-year-old could expect to live to 148. Drugs of this sort may have been in use since sometime before 2030. A drug resulting

Figure 12-3. Effect of Anti-Aging Substances

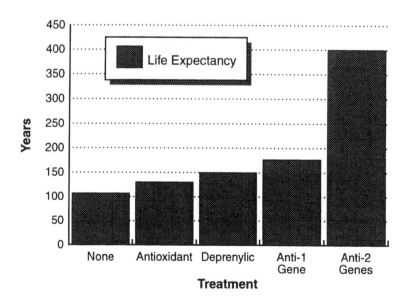

from the extension of current research on deprenyl or dietary restriction is also likely to be in use by 2050 and would raise life expectancy to about 150. A 35-year-old could expect to live to 170.

By 2050, research on the genes that control aging should have found drugs that block at least some of these genes in laboratory animals and human cells grown in culture. Human testing will likely be underway. These drugs, plus further advances in medicine, will promise a truly astounding rise in longevity in the years ahead.

Life Extension In 2080

Barring a global catastrophe, the world of 2080 will be as far beyond the world of 2000 as the world of 2000 is beyond the world of 1800. Those 80 years of advances will easily equal the 200 years of progress before the year 2000. The state of technology in the world of 2080 is beyond the scope of our discussion, but I suspect the world of 2080 will be almost unrecognizable to someone from 2000.

Thirty years of rapid progress beyond the advanced state of medicine of 2050 should see us able to prevent or cure 90 percent of all diseases. We should control almost all infectious diseases. Many will have already vanished. Gene therapy should erase hereditary diseases and the surprisingly large number of diseases having a genetic predisposition. Prevention, monitoring, computerized medicine, organ replacement (cloned and artificial), and strong immunity will virtually abolish deaths from disease. Injuries will occur. If needed, the replacement of organs and most body parts may be as routine as replacing the parts of an automobile. Sporadically, a new infectious disease will flare up to cause deaths and spur a flurry of research before we conquer it. Accidents will probably continue to be the leading cause of death, but high-tech safety measures should reduce accidental deaths to 25 percent of those in 2000.

By 2080, researchers should know all the details of

aging and its control. Drugs blocking aging genes will have passed decades of experimental development, testing on human volunteers, and FDA approval. They should control some, and likely all, of the genes that cause aging. They may not be totally effective, but they should slow aging to a crawl.

The conquest of 90 percent of diseases will contribute to a further rise in the life expectancy of health-conscious persons who use all methods of prevention and cure in 2080. From only the conquest of diseases,

- Life expectancy at birth will be 113 years.
- A 35-year-old can expect to live to 130.
- A 100-year-old can expect to live to 145.
- Someone born in 1920 may reach a maximum life span of 160.

But the big extension of life should come from blocking the genes that cause aging. Even incomplete control of the genes should cause an astounding rise in longevity. If humans have counterparts of age-1, daf-2, or clk-1, blocking one should increase the life expectancy of health-conscious persons to approximately 180 years. A 35-year-old could expect to live to 200. If two can be blocked, it may extend life expectancy right on past 300 to almost 500 years. After 2080, it is likely that research will move quickly to change the genes that cause aging. This will stop the aging process permanently. At the same time, research will continue to conquer the few diseases that remain.

Life Extension In 2100

It is not feasible to imagine what life will be like in 2100. If we extrapolate from 1790 to 1990, we may get a feeling of how life may be—computerized, served by robots, with unlimited sources of power, and incredibly advanced. It may be a more civilized and happier place than today, with more time for art, music, and literature. Unless our brains become mushy in the intervening years, it probably will. People in 2100 may look back on 1990 somewhat as we today look back on the Dark Ages.

Medicine will have advanced for a century beyond the medicine of 2000. Knowledge of the workings of the body, even the tiniest details about the activity of every protein in living cells, should be complete. We should be able to prevent or cure 95 percent, and probably 99 percent, of all diseases. Death from diseases should be rare. Aside from keeping people's bodies working smoothly, the major task of medicine may be repairing injuries from accidents or foul play. To permit rapid repair, cloned or artificial versions of every part of the body—even the most obscure—will be available.

Continued research on the control of the genes that cause aging should result in a permanent halt to aging by

Figure 12-4. Projected Longevity

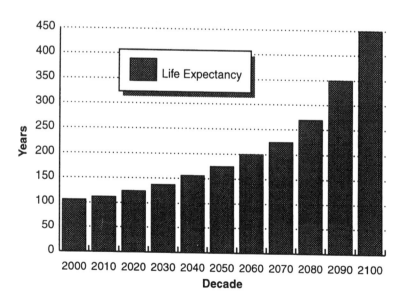

gene therapy. Genes responsible for the replacement of proteins and the repair of cell structures should switch on permanently.

The unthinkable will also become permanent. By restoring protein synthesis and other cellular activities to their levels in young cells, the cells will become young again. A person with young cells is physically young, regardless of age. Thus, we not only will stop persons from aging, we also will reverse it. This will give you an indefinite life span in a youthful body. Your life span will be open ended. A person who maintains health and avoids falling into an active volcano can look forward to living hundreds of years.

Figure 12-4 shows the projected rise in life expectancy of health-conscious persons. Life expectancy in 2000 is about 100 years, depending on one's age. The climb is slow in the early decades of the twenty-first century but accelerates as the influence of controlling aging becomes progressively larger. By 2100, we are looking at indefinite longevity, limited mainly by accidents.

Will we do it? We began our look at life extension with a perceptive observation by Arthur Clarke: *Anything that is theoretically possible will be achieved in practice, no matter what the technical difficulties, if it is desired greatly enough.*

This has been true for hundreds of advances. Provided they can be healthy and active, most people will want very much to live as long as possible. We will do it. People in 2100 will look back and snicker at those who declared we couldn't.

A Timetable For Longevity

Let's see how all of this may affect you. A health-conscious person born in 1990, who avoids accidents or violence, should live on past 2100. But let's assume you were 65 in 1990. You are health-conscious and follow a program of preventive medicine. You do not smoke and avoid secondhand smoke. You exercise daily. You eat a balanced, low-fat diet with a high proportion of fresh fruits and vegetables. You keep your weight in the optimum range. You have a thorough medical exam yearly by an up-to-date internist. You immunize against pneumonia, influenza, and other infectious diseases. You act to avoid accidents and violence. These actions can help you reach 2000.

By 2000, you will be 75. Since you are health-conscious, your life expectancy will be 105. You can expect to live to 2030. The period between 2000 and 2030 will be your most perilous as advances in medicine fight to keep you ahead of diseases, a lowered immune system, and the devastation of aging.

By 2030, you will be 105. Your future looks hopeful. With the further conquest of diseases, your life expectancy should rise to 117. The most important event for you is the arrival of the first drugs to slow aging. They should raise your life expectancy at least 20 percent. You can expect to live to 140, which you will reach in 2065.

By 2050, you will be 125 years old. You are nearly there! An anti-aging drug has you feeling and acting much like a 45-year-old. We should have overcome half the diseases that killed us in 1990. Your immune system is fully functional, so the threat of disease is fading. From the reduction in diseases alone, your life expectancy would only be 125, but drugs to control the genes that cause aging will raise this further. As a result, you can expect to live to 175, which you will reach at the dawn of the new millennium in 2100.

By 2080, you will be 155. It's in the bag now! We should have virtually eliminated deaths from diseases. This will raise life expectancy to 130. But the drugs to block genes involved in aging, although not completely effective, will push your life span to 260, which you will reach in 2185. You also look, feel, and act like a young adult.

By 2100, you will be 175. By then we should be able to

prevent or cure almost any disease. Gene therapy has stopped you from aging permanently. You can expect to live indefinitely in your youthful body, unless you run afoul of accident, violence, or an unknown disease. You can sit back with a cold drink and contemplate all the things you have done, and all the things you are going to do: the places you will go, the people you will meet, the music, art, entertainment, reading, travel, adventure, and everything else you want to do. You will have time for it—plenty of time.

If you were younger than 65 in 1990, your chances are even better, provided that you also survive the perilous time between now and 2030.

Of course, there are no guarantees. All of this assumes that research continues at its present rate and that no global disasters involving fanatics with nuclear weapons, the depletion of the ozone layer, the greenhouse effect, collisions with asteroids, or other horrors befall us. It also assumes that you survive the near future, from now to 2030, the period when the chance of being killed by diseases is greatest.

If you are health-conscious, from now on, each year you survive will raise your chance of living longer. It's a sparkling future, and we're speeding into it at 1,000 miles per hour.

Appendix

How To Estimate Your Longevity

Nothing is guaranteed in this world, but we have seen many things you can do today that will probably extend your healthy, active life. The following list contains known actions that can extend your life, so add them up and see how you are doing. As a basis, figure the average life expectancy at birth today is 76. If you are now 35, you can expect to live to 78. If you are 65, you can expect to live to 82.

Some of the actions may prevent other diseases and extend your life expectancy further. These are only estimates to give you a feeling for what you can accomplish. Many factors can influence them. The discovery of new preventive measures will raise the estimates. The first drug to control aging will send them sky high.

ACTION	ADD
No smoking	9 years
Exercise and sleep	3 years
Good diet, desirable weight, (cholesterol-lowering drugs, estrogen)	3 years
Daily aspirin	1 year
Thorough medical exam yearly	2 years

Prevent hypertension	1 year
Avoid accidents	1 year
Immunize against pneumonia/influenza	1 year
Avoid suicide and AIDS	1 year
Avoid heavy alcohol consumption	1 year

How are these additions to life expectancy estimated? Life expectancy is the product of a series of calculations based on death rate at each age in a population, from newborn to very old. The population can be that of a nation or that of a group of people (health-conscious individuals, for example). The calculation is such that anything reducing the death rate automatically raises life expectancy. For example, not smoking reduces deaths from cardiovascular disease by almost 50 percent, cancer by 44 percent, stroke by 50 percent, and chronic lung disease by 85 percent. Since these are the four main causes of death, not smoking decreases overall deaths sharply and boosts life expectancy by many years.

References

Introduction

Clark, A.C., *Profiles of the Future*. Harper and Row, New York (1963).

Sagan, C., *The Demon-Haunted World: Science as a candle in the dark*. Random House, New York (1995).

Chapter 1 — Thinking The Unthinkable

Acsadi, G. and Nemeskeri, J., *History of Human Life Span and Mortality*. Academiai Kiado, Budapest (1970).

Bennett, N.G. and Garson, L.K., Extraordinary longevity in the Soviet Union: fact or artifact? *Gerontologist* 26, 358 (1986).

Bortz, W.M., *We Live Too Short and Die Too Long*. Bantam, New York (1991).

Hall, S.S., How technique is changing science. *Science* 257, 344 (1992).

Iglehart, J.K., Medical care of the poor — a growing problem. *New England Journal of Medicine* 313, 59 (1985).

MacDonnell, W.R., On the expectation of life in ancient Rome and in the provinces of Hispania and Lusitania, and Africa. *Biometrika* 9, 366 (1913).

Mazess, R.B. and Forman, S.H., Longevity and age exaggeration in Vilcabamba, Ecuador. *Journal of Gerontology* 34, 94 (1979).

at how fast we have progressed. In 1975 we had growing evidence that genes control longevity, but we had no idea what genes are involved. We were occupied with discovering how aging changes activities inside cells. By 1985, researchers were identifying genes whose expression fell in old age. Most retained 10-50 percent of their activity, indicating the fall in expression resulted from the loss of a transcription factor. By 1995, the number of genes known to switch off partially had grown rapidly. Researchers had found that senescent cells switch off several of their regulator genes that each control large groups of genes. Of enormous importance was the discovery of genes that control longevity. Age-1, daf-2, and LAG 1 are genes in simple organisms. But the finding of similar genes in mammalian and human cells indicates that age-1, daf-2, and clk-1 will lead us to the genes controlling human longevity. Considering that the control of genes that govern longevity will eliminate aging, the advances between 1985 and 1995 were immense.

All evidence points to even greater advances in coming years. We should identify the genes that control longevity in simple organisms. We should use not only LAG 1, but also age-1, daf-2, and similar genes to find out whether they have counterparts in mammals and humans. We should know whether these genes cause senescence by producing suppressors of regulator genes or whether they act in some other way. We may also know whether there is a longevity gene that keeps senescence genes suppressed until old age and how telomere length, or another mechanism, controls it.

Beyond 2005, as we learn still more about the genes that cause aging, the search will likely be for ways to control aging and extend longevity for many years. Although centrophenoxine is an unlikely candidate, we may find other drugs that block the action of senescence genes. These might include antisense DNA, but the problem of *bled the life span of the human cells.* More treatment with antisense DNA might have extended the lifespan further. This is an important finding, not because antisense DNA for this mRNA will extend life but because it shows a way to control senescence genes by binding the mRNA they produce. First, we must identify senescence genes (like the human equivalent of age-1) whose mRNAs must be tied up. Second, we must be able to deliver antisense DNAs into our cells. Then, regular treatment with antisense DNAs could extend life indefinitely.

Finally, we could insert longevity genes into cells under independent control. The first two means to halt aging employ a drug or antisense DNA. These methods would require you to take a capsule or an injection regularly. The ideal situation is to halt aging permanently. Researchers have already advanced toward this goal. One group has taken genes for an elongation protein (which helps ribosomes make proteins) and has altered their control regions so that they are permanently switched on. Inserted into fruit flies, they slowed aging and caused the maximum lifespan to rise 42 percent. If the same technique worked in health-conscious humans, it could raise life expectancy to nearly 150 years and the maximum life span to 170 years. Another group has inserted into fruit flies additional copies of genes for proteins that protect against oxidation. The maximum life span rose 34 percent.

These effects came from the insertion of cellular genes. What might happen if we were to insert longevity genes? In the scheme outlined above, insertion of longevity genes into protected areas of chromosomes could, barring disease or an accident, extend life indefinitely. At the rate gene therapy is advancing, this should be possible by the time we identify the genes that cause aging.

The Road Ahead

To get a sense of what is ahead, we should look back

Guiness Book of World Records. Bantam, New York (1989).

Mee, C.L., Medieval Europe and the killer fleas. *Smithsonian* 20, 66 (1990).

National Center for Health Statistics, *Advance Report of Final Mortality Statistics, 1990.* Hyattsville, MD, U.S. Dept. of Health and Human Services (1993).

Pifer, A. and Bronte, L. (eds.), *Our Aging Society: Paradox and Promise.* Norton, New York (1986).

Vallois, H.V., La duree de vie chez l'homme fossile. *Comptes Rendus Academie Sciences* 204, 60 (1937).

Chapter 2 — The Conquest Of Cardiovascular Disease

Austen, W.G. and Cosimi, A.B., Heart transplantation after 16 years. *New England Journal of Medicine* 311, 1436 (1984).

Blankenhorn, D.H., Johnson, R.L., Mack, W.J., El Zein, H.A., and Vailas, L.I., The influence of diet on the appearance of new lesions in human coronary arteries. *Journal of the American Medical Association* 263, 1646 (1990).

Bradford, R.H., Shear, C.L., Chremos, A.N., and coworkers, Expanded clinical evaluation of lovastatin (EXCEL) study results. I. Efficiency in modifying plasma lipoproteins and adverse event profile in 8,245 patients with moderate hypercholesterolemia. *Archives of Internal Medicine* 151, 43 (1991).

Bradford, R.H., Downton, M., Chremos, A.N., and coworkers, Efficacy and tolerability of Lovastatin in 3390 women with moderate hypercholesterolemia. *Archives of Internal Medicine* 118, 851 (1993).

Brown, G., Albers, J.J., Fisher, L.D., and coworkers, Regression of coronary artery disease as a result of intensive lipid-lowering therapy in men with high levels of apolipoprotein B. *New England Journal of Medicine* 323, 1289 (1990).

Brown, M.S. and Goldstein, J.L., Heart attacks: gone with the century? *Science* 272, 629 (1996).

Burke, G.L., Sprafka, J.M., and coworkers, Trends in serum cholesterol from 1980 to 1987. *New England Journal of Medicine* 324, 941 (1991).

Chowdhury, J.R., Grossman, M., Gupta, S., and coworkers, Long-term improvement of hypercholesterolemia after ex vivo gene therapy in LDLR-deficient rabbits. *Science* 254, 1802 (1991).

Cohn, J.N. and 18 others, A comparison of enalapril and hydralazine-isosorbide dinitrate in the treatment of chronic congestive heart failure. *New England Journal of Medicine* 325, 303 (1991).

Enstrom, J.E., Health practices and cancer mortality among active California Mormons. *Journal of the National Cancer Institute* 81, 1807 (1989).

Enstrom, J.E., Kanim, L.E., and Klein, M.A., Vitamin C intake and mortality among a sample of the United States population. *Epidemiology* 3, 194 (1992).

Feldman, A.M. and the Vesnarinone Research Group, Effect of Vesnarinone on morbidity and mortality of patients with heart failure. *New England Journal of Medicine* 329, 1 (1993).

Fielding, J.E., Smoking: health effects and control. *New England Journal of Medicine* 313, 491 (1985).

Fisher, J.A., *Rx 2000: Breakthroughs in Health, Medicine, and Longevity by the Year 2000 and Beyond.* Simon and Schuster, New York (1992).

Gey, E.F., Pekka, P., Jordan, P., and Moser, U.K., Inverse correlation between plasma vitamin E and mortality from ischemic heart disease in cross-cultural epidemiology. *American Journal of Clinical Nutrition* 53, 326S (1991).

Goy, J.J., Sigwart, U., Vogt, P., and coworkers, Long term follow-up of the first 56 patients treated with intra-coronary self-expanding stents (the Lausanne experience). *American Journal of Cardiology* 67, 569 (1991).

Guralnik, J.M. and Kaplan, G.A., Predictors of healthy aging: prospective evidence from the Alameda County Study. *American Journal of Public Health* 79, 703 (1989).

Hubert, H.B., Feinleib, M., McNamara, P.M., and Castelli, W.P., Obesity as an independent risk factor for cardiovascular disease: a 26-year followup of participants in the Framingham Heart Study. *Circulation* 67, 968 (1983).

Kane, J.P., Malloy, M.J., Ports, T.A., and coworkers, Regression of coronary atherosclerosis during treatment of familial hypercholesterolemia with combined drug regimens. *Journal of the American Medical Association* 264, 3007 (1990).

Kennedy, J.W., Ritchie, J.L., Davis, K.B., and coworkers, The western Washington randomized trial of intracoronary streptokinase in acute myocardial infarction. *New England Journal of Medicine* 312, 1073 (1985).

King, A.C., Frey-Hewitt, B., Dreon, D., and Wood, P.D., Diet vs exercise in weight maintenance: the effects of minimal intervention strategies on long-term outcomes in men. *Archives of Internal Medicine* 149, 2741 (1989).

Kuczmarski, R.J., Flegal, K.M., Campbell, S.M., and Johnson, C.L., Increasing prevalence of overweight among U.S. adults. *Journal of the American Medical Association* 272, 205 (1994).

LaCroix, A.Z., Lang, J., Scherr, P., and coworkers, Smoking and mortality among older men and women in three communities. *New England Journal of Medicine* 324, 1619 (1991).

Lefer, A,M., Tsao, P., Aoki, N., and Palladino, Jr., M.A., Mediation of cardioprotection by transforming growth factor-beta. *Science* 249, 61 (1990).

Machlin, L.J. and Bendich, A., Free radical tissue damage: protective role of antioxidant nutrients. *FASEB Journal* 1, 441 (1987).

Manson, J.E., Colditz, G.A., Stampfer, H.J., and coworkers, A prospective study of obesity and risk of coronary heart disease in women. *New England Journal of Medicine* 322, 882 (1990).

Manson, J.E., Willett, W.C., Stampfer, M.J., and coworkers, Body weight and mortality among women. *New England Journal of Medicine* 333, 677 (1995).

Manson, J., Stampfer, M., Colditz, G., and coworkers, A prospective study of aspirin use and prevention of cardiovascular disease in women. *Journal of the American Medical Association* 266, 521 (1991).

National Center for Health Statistics, *Vital Statistics of the United States, 1988. Life Tables.* DHHS, Hyattsville, MD (1991).

Ornish, D., *Doctor Dean Ornish's Program for Reducing Heart Disease.* Random House, New York (1990).

Paffenbarger, R.S., Hyde, R.T., and Wing, A.L., Physical activity, all-cause mortality, and longevity of college alumni. *New England Journal of Medicine* 314, 605 (1986).

Rimm, E.B., Stampfer, M.J., Ascherio, A., and coworkers, Vitamin E consumption and the risk of coronary heart disease in men. *New England Journal of Medicine* 328, 1450 (1993).

Rosenberg, L., Kaufman, D.W., Helmrich, S.P., and Shapiro, S., The risk of myocardial infarction after quitting smoking in men under 55 years of age. *New England Journal of Medicine* 313, 1511 (1985).

Segerberg, O.Jr., *Living to be 100*. New York, Scribners (1982).

Stampfer, M.J., Sacks, F.M., Salvini, S., Willett, W.C., and Hennekens, C.H., A prospective study of cholesterol, apolipoproteins, and the risk of myocardial infarction. *New England Journal of Medicine* 325, 373 (1991).

Stampfer, M.J., Colditz, G.A., Willett, W.C., and coworkers, Postmenopausal estrogen therapy and cardiovascular disease. *New England Journal of Medicine* 325, 756 (1991).

Stampfer, M.J., Hennekens, C.H., Manson, J.E., and coworkers, Vitamin E consumption and the risk of coronary disease in women. *New England Journal of Medicine* 328, 1444 (1993).

Surgeon General, *The Health Consequences of Smoking: Cardiovascular Disease. A Report of the Surgeon General.* DHHS, Rockville, MD (1983).

Surgeon General, *The Health Consequences of Involuntary Smoking: A Report.* DHHS, Rockville, MD (1984).

Sytkowski, P.A., Kannel, W.B., and D'Agostino, R.B., Changes in risk factors and the decline in mortality from cardiovascular disease. The Framingham Heart Study. *New England Journal of Medicine* 322, 1635 (1990).

Timmis, A.D., Early diagnosis of acute myocardial infarction. *British Medical Journal* 301, 941 (1990).

Veith, F.J., Bakal, C.W., Cynamon, J., and coworkers, Early experience with the smart laser in the treatment of atherosclerotic occlusions. *American Heart Journal* 121, 1531 (1990).

Wannamethee, G. and Shaper, A.G., Body weight and mortality in middle aged British men: impact of smoking. *British Medical Journal* 299, 1497 (1989).

Warner, K.E., The economics of smoking: dollars and sense. *New York State Journal of Medicine* 83, 1273 (1983).

Willett, W.G., Green, A., Stampfer, M.J., and coworkers, Relative and absolute excess risks of coronary heart disease among women who smoke cigarettes. *New England Journal of Medicine* 317, 1303 (1987).

Yanagisawa-Miwa, A., Uchida, Y., Nakamura, F., and coworkers, Salvage of infarcted myocardium by angiogenic action of basic fibroblast growth factor. *Science* 257, 1401 (1992).

Chapter 3 — Progress Against Cancer

Baker, S.J., Markowitz, S., Fearon, E.R., Willson, J.K.V., and Vogelstein, B., Suppression of human colorectal carcinoma cell growth by wild-type p53. *Science* 249, 912 (1990).

Balducci, L., Practical screening for malignancy. *Hospital Medicine* 27, 44 (1991).

Benedict, W.F., Wheatley, W.L., and Jones, P.A., Inhibition of chemically induced morphological transformation and reversion of the transformed phenotype by ascorbic acid in C3H/10T-1/2 cells. *Cancer Research* 40, 2796 (1980).

Block, G., Vitamin C and cancer prevention: the epidemiologic evidence. *American Journal of Clinical Nutrition* 53, 270S (1991).

Boring, C.C., Squires, T.S., and Tong, T., Cancer statistics, 1991. *Ca - A Cancer Journal for Clinicians* 41, 19 (1991).

Callahan, R. and Campbell, G., Mutations in human breast cancer: an overview. *Journal of the National Cancer Institute* 81, 1780 (1989).

Catalona, W.J., Smith, D.S., Ratleff, T.L., and coworkers, Measurement of prostate-specific antigen in serum as a screening test for prostate cancer. *New England Journal of Medicine* 324, 1156 (1991).

Chen, P.L., Chen, Y., Bookstein, R., and Lee, W.H., Genetic mechanisms of tumor suppression by the human p53 gene. *Science* 250, 1576 (1990).

Comstock, G.W., Helzlsouer, K.J., and Bush, T.L., Prediagnostic serum levels of carotenoids and vitamin E as related to subsequent cancer in Washington County, Maryland. *American Journal of Clinical Nutrition* 53, 260S (1991).

Cook, M.G. and McNamara, P., Effect of dietary vitamin E on dimethylhydrazine-induced colonic tumors. *Cancer Research* 40, 1329 (1980).

Doll, R. and Peto, R., *The Causes of Cancer.* Oxford University Press (1981).

Fisher, J.A., *Rx 2000: Breakthroughs in Health, Medicine, and Longevity by the Year 2000 and Beyond.* Simon and Schuster, New York (1992).

Gardner, J.W. and Lyon, J.L., Cancer in Utah Mormon men by lay priesthood level. *American Journal of Epidemiology* 116, 243 (1982).

Garfinkel, L. and Silverberg, E., Lung cancer and smoking trends in the United States over the past 25 years. *CA - A Cancer Journal For Clinicians* 41, 137 (1991).

Golumber, P.T., Lazenby, A.J., Levitsky, H.I., and coworkers, Treatment of established renal cancer by tumor cells engineered to secrete Interleukin-4. *Science* 254, 713 (1991).

Greenberg, E.R. and coworkers, A clinical trial of beta-carotene to prevent basal-cell and squamous-cell cancers of the skin. *New England Journal of Medicine* 323, 789 (1990).

Heinonen, O.P., Albanes, D., and the Alpha-Tocopherol, Beta-Carotene Cancer Prevention Study Group, The effect of vitamin E and beta carotene on the incidence of lung cancer and other cancers in male smokers. *New England Journal of Medicine* 330, 1029 (1994).

Henderson, B.E., Ross, R.K., and Pike, M.C., Toward the primary prevention of cancer. *Science* 254, 1131 (1991).

Horvath, P.M. and Ip, C., Synergistic effect of vitamin E and selenium in the chemoprevention of mammary carcinogenesis in rats. *Cancer Research* 43, 5335 (1983).

Knekt, P., Aromaa, A., Maatela, J., and coworkers, Vitamin E and cancer prevention. *American Journal of Clinical Nutrition* 53, 283S (1991).

Kolonel, L.N., Nomura, A.M., Hirohata, Y., and coworkers, Association of diet and place of birth with stomach cancer incidence in Hawaii Japanese and Caucasians. *American Journal of Clinical Nutrition* 34, 2478 (1980).

Krinsky, N.I., Carotenoids and cancer in animal models. *Journal of Nutrition* 119, 123 (1989).

LaCroix, A.Z., Lang, J., Scherr, P., and coworkers, Smoking and mortality among older men and women in three communities. *New England Journal of Medicine* 324, 1619 (1991).

Lundberg, G., In developed countries, the golden age of medicine is at hand — for the patients. *Journal of the American Medical Association,* 258, 2415 (1987).

Martuza, R.L., Malick, A., Markert, J.R., Ruffner, K.L., and Coen, D.M.,, Experimental therapy of human glioma by means of a genetically engineered virus mutant. *Science* 252, 854 (1991).

Menck, H.R., Garfinkel, L., and Dodd, G.D., Preliminary report of the National Cancer Data Base. *Ca - A Cancer Journal for Clinicians* 41, 7 (1991).

Menkes, M.S., Comstock, G.W., Vuilleumier, J.P., and coworkers, Serum beta-carotene, vitamins A and E, selenium, and the risk of lung cancer. *New England Journal of Medicine* 315, 1250 (1986).

Moon, R.C., Comparative aspects of carotenoids and retinoids as chemopreventive agents for cancer. *Journal of Nutrition* 119, 127 (1989).

Nicolaou, K.C., Dai, W.M., Tsay, S.C., Estevez, V.A., and Wrasidlo, W., Designed enediynes: A new class of DNA-cleaving molecules with potent and selective anticancer activity. *Science* 256, 1172 (1992).

Repace, J.L. and Lowrey, A.H., A quantitative estimate of nonsmokers lung cancer risk from passive smoking. *Environment International* 11, 3 (1985).

Selby, J.V. and Friedman, G.D., U.S. preventive services task force: sigmoidoscopy in the periodic health examination of asymptomatic adults. *Journal of the American Medical Association* 261, 594 (1989).

Shamberger, R.J., Relationship of selenium to cancer. I. Inhibitory effect of selenium on carcinogenesis. *Journal of the National Cancer Institute* 44, 931 (1970).

Stevens, R.G., Jones, D.Y., Micozzi, M.S., and Taylor, P.R., Body iron stores and the risk of cancer. *New England Journal of Medicine* 319, 1047 (1988).

Surgeon General, *The Health Consequences of Smoking. Cancer, a Report of the Surgeon General.* DHHS, Rockville, MD (1982).

Szczylik, C., Skorski, T., Nicolaides, N.C., and coworkers, Selective inhibition of leukemia cell proliferation by BCR-ABL antisense ologonucleotides. *Science* 253, 562 (1991).

Thun, M.J., Namboodiri, M.M., and Heath, Jr., C.W., Aspirin use and reduced risk of fatal colon cancer. *New England Journal of Medicine* 325, 1593 (1991).

Trail, P.A., Willner, D., and coworkers, Cure of xenografted human carcinomas by BR96-doxorubicin immunoconjugates. *Science* 261, 212 (1993).

Trauth, B.C., Klas, C., Peters, A.M., and coworkers, Monoclonal antibody-mediated tumor regression by induction of apoptosis. *Science* 245, 301 (1989).

Trichopoulos, D., Mollo, F., Tomatis, L., and coworkers, Active and passive smoking and pathological indicators of lung cancer risk in an autopsy study. *Journal of the American Medical Association* 268, 1697 (1992).

Trojan, J., Johnson, T.R., Rudin, S.D., and coworkers, Treatment and prevention of rat glioblastoma by immunogenic C6 cells expressing antisense insulin-like growth factor-1 RNA. *Science* 259, 94 (1993).

Whittemore, A.S., Wu-Williams, A.H., Lee, M., and coworkers, K., Diet, physical activity, and colorectal cancer among Chinese in North America and China. *Journal of the National Cancer Institute* 82, 915 (1990).

Willett, W.G., Stampfer, M.J., Colditz, G.A., and coworkers, Relation of meat, fat, and fiber to the risk of colon cancer. *New England Journal of Medicine* 323, 1664 (1990).

Ziegler, R.G., A review of epidemiologic evidence that carotenoids reduce the risk of cancer. *Journal of Nutrition* 119, 116 (1989).

Chapter 4 — Extending Life Beyond 100

Abbott, R.D., Yin Yin, M.A., Reed, D.M., and Yano, K., Risk of stroke in male cigarette smokers. *New England Journal of Medicine* 315, 717 (1986).

Bendich, A., Gabriel, E., and Machlin, L.J., Dietary vitamin E requirement for optimum immune responses in the rat. *Journal of Nutrition* 116, 675 (1986).

Chilmonszyk, B.A., Salmun, L.M., Megathlin, K.N., and co-workers, Association between exposure to environmental tobacco smoke and exascerbation of asthma in children. *New England Journal of Medicine* 328, 1665 (1993).

Ebright, J.R. and Rytel, M.W., Bacterial pneumonia in the elderly. *Journal of the American Geriatrics Society* 28, 220 (1980).

Faustman, D. and Coe, C., Prevention of xenograft rejection by masking donor HLA Class I antigens. *Science* 252, 1700 (1991).

Fisher, M. and Bougasslavsky, J., Evolving toward effective therapy for acute ischemic strokes. *Journal of the American Medical Association* 270, 360 (1993).

Gill, J.S., Zezulka, J.V., Shipley, M.J., and coworkers, Stroke and alcohol consumption. *New England Journal of Medicine* 315, 1041 (1986).

Helmrich, S.P., Rayland, D.R., Leung, R.W., and Paffenberger, R.S., Physical activity and reduced occurrence of non-insulin-dependent diabetes mellitus. *New England Journal of Medicine* 325, 147 (1991).

Kellerman, A.L., et al., Suicide in the home in relation to gun ownership. *New England Journal of Medicine* 327, 467 (1992).

Khaw, K.T. and Barrett-Connor, E., Dietary potassium and stroke-associated mortality. *New England Journal of Medicine* 316, 235 (1987).

Lacy, P.E., Hegre, O.D., Gerasimidi-Vazeou, A., and coworkers, Maintenance of normoglycemia in diabetic mice by subcutaneous xenografts of encapsulated islets. *Science* 254, 1782 (1991).

Makinodan, T. and Albright, J.W., Restoration of impaired immune functions in aging animals. *Mechanisms of Ageing and Development* 11, 1 (1979).

Meydani, S.N., Barklund, M.P., Liu, S., and coworkers, Vitamin E supplementation enhances cell-mediated immunity in healthy elderly subjects. *American Journal of Clinical Nutrition* 52, 557 (1990).

Shapiro, E.D., Berg, A.T., Austrian, R., and coworkers, The protective efficacy of polyvalent pneumococcal polysaccharide vaccine. *New England Journal of Medicine* 325, 1453 (1991).

Surgeon General, *The Health Consequences of Smoking: Chronic Obstructive Lung Disease. A Report of the Surgeon General.* DHHS, Rockville, MD (1984).

Chapter 5 — Your Inner Longevity Factor

Beecher, H.K., The powerful placebo. *Journal of the American Medical Association* 159, 1602 (1955).

Benson, H., *The Mind/Body Effect.* Simon and Schuster, New York (1979).

Calabrese, J.R., Kling, M.A., and Gold, P.W., Alterations in immunocompetence during stress, bereavement, and depression. *American Journal of Psychiatry* 144, 1123 (1987).

Cassileth, B.R., Lusk, E.J., Miller, D.S., Brown, L.L., and Miller, C., Psychosocial correlates of survival in advanced malignant disease? *New England Journal of Medicine* 312, 368 (1985).

Cousins, N., *Anatomy of an Illness.* Norton, New York (1979).

Cousins, N., *Head First. The Biology of Hope and the Healing Power of the Human Spirit.* Penguin, New York (1989).

Derogatis, L.R., Abeloff, M.D., and Melisaratos, N., Psychological coping mechanisms and survival time in metastatic breast cancer. *Journal of the American Medical Association* 242, 1504 (1979).

Friedman, M., Rosenman, R.H., and Carroll, V., Changes in serum cholesterol and blood clotting time in men subjected to cyclic variation in occupational stress. *Circulation* 17, 852 (1958).

Glaser, R, Kiecolt-Glaser, J.K., Stout, J.C., and coworkers, Stress-related impairments in cellular immunity. *Psychiatry Research* 16, 233 (1985).

Kiecolt-Glaser, J.K., Glaser, R., Williger, D., and coworkers, Psychosocial enhancement of immunocompetence in a geriatric population. *Health Psychology* 4, 24 (1985).

Locke, S. and Colligan, D., *The Healer Within: The New Medicine of Mind and Body.* Dutton, New York (1986).

Ross, S. and Buckalew, L., The placebo as an agent of behavioral manipulation. *Clinical Psychology* Review 3, 457 (1983).

Rozanski, A., Bairey, C.N., Krantz, D.S., and coworkers, Mental stress in the induction of silent myocardial ischemia in patients with coronary artery disease. *New England Journal of Medicine* 318, 1005 (1988).

Selye, H. *The Stress of Life.* McGraw-Hill, New York (1956).

Solomon, G.F., Fiatarone, M.A., Benton, D., and coworkers, Psychoimmunologic and endorphin function in the aged. *Annals of the New York Academy of Sciences* 521, 42 (1988).

Chapter 6 — How Far Can Medicine Go?

Bendich, A., Gabriel, E., and Machlin, L.J., Dietary vitamin E requirement for optimum immune response in the rat. *Journal of Nutrition* 116, 675 (1986).

Davis, K.L., Thal, L.J., Gamzu, E.R., and the Tacrine Collaborative Study Group, A double-blind, placebo-controlled multi-center study of Tacrine for Alzheimer's disease. *New England Journal of Medicine* 327, 1253 (1992).

Esch, F.S., Keim, P.S., Beattie, E.C., and coworkers, Cleavage of amyloid beta peptide during constituitive processing of its precursor. *Science* 248, 1122 (1990).

Evans, D.A., Funkstein, D.H., Albert, M.S., and coworkers, Prevalence of Alzheimer's disease in a community population of older persons. *Journal of the American Medical Association* 262, 2551 (1989).

Farlow, M., Gracon, S.I., Hershey, L.A., and the Tacrine Study Group, A controlled trial of Tacrine in Alzheimer's disease. *Journal of the American Medical Association* 268, 2523 (1992).

Golde, T.E., Estus, S., Younkin, L.H., and coworkers, Processing the amyloid protein precursor to potentially amyloidogenic derivatives. *Science* 255, 728 (1992).

Katzman, R., Alzheimer's disease. *New England Journal of Medicine* 314, 964 (1986).

Katzman, R. and Saitoh, T., Advances in Alzheimer's disease. *FASEB Journal* 5, 278 (1991).

Kohn, R.R., Causes of death in very old people. *Journal of the American Medical Association* 247, 2793 (1982).

Manton, K.G., Cause specific mortality patterns among the oldest old: multiple cause of death trends 1968 to 1980. *Journal of Gerontology* 41, 282 (1986).

Manton, K.G., Past and future life expectancy increases at later ages: their implications for the linkage of chronic morbidity, disability, and mortality. *Journal of Gerontology* 41, 672 (1986).

Murrell, J., Farlow, M., Ghetti, B., and Benson, M., A mutation in the amyloid precursor protein associated with hereditary Alzheimer's disease. *Science* 254, 97 (1991).

Olshansky, S.J., Carnes, B.A., and Cassel, C., In search of Methuselah: estimating the upper limits of human longevity. *Science* 250, 634 (1990).

Rosenberg, B., Kemeny, G., Smith, L.G., Skurnick, I.D., and Bandurski, M.J., The kinetics and thermodynamics of death in multicellular organisms. *Mechanisms of Ageing and Development*, 2, 275-294 (1973).

Schellenberg, G.D., Bird, T.D., Wijsman, E.M., and coworkers, Genetic linkage evidence for a familial Alzheimer's disease locus on chromosome 14. *Science* 258, 668 (1992).

Scinto, L.F.M., Daffner, K.R., Dressler, D., and coworkers, A potential noninvasive neurobiological test for Alzheimer's disease. *Science* 266, 1051 (1994).

Sisodia, S.S., Koo, E.H., Beyreuther, K., Unterbeck, A., and Price, D.L., Evidence that beta-amyloid protein in Alzheimer's disease is not derived by normal processing. *Science* 248, 492 (1990).

Spittle, C.R., The action of vitamin C on blood vessels. *American Heart Journal* 88, 387 (1974).

Trentham, D.E., Dynesius-Trentham, R.A., Orav, E.J., and coworkers, Effects of oral administration of Type II collagen on rheumatoid arthritis. *Science* 261, 1727 (1993).

Watts, N.B., and coworkers, Intermittent cyclical etidronate treatment of postmenopausal osteoporosis. *New England Journal of Medicine* 323, 73 (1990).

Yankner, B., Dawes, L., Fisher, S., and coworkers, Neurotoxicity of a fragment of the amyloid precursor associated with Alzheimer's disease. *Science* 245, 417 (1989).

Chapter 7 — What We Know About Aging

Brandfonbrenner, M., Landowne, M., and Shock, N.W., Changes in cardiac output with age. *Circulation* 12, 567 (1955).

Comfort, A., *The Biology of Senescence*. 3rd Edition. Elsevier, New York (1979).

Davies, D.F. and Shock, N.W., Age changes in glomerular filtration rate, effective renal plasma flow, and tubular excretory capacity in adult males. *Journal of Clinical Investigation* 29, 496 (1950).

Dehn, M.M. and Bruce, R.A., Longitudinal variations in maximal oxygen uptake decreases uniformly from childhood throughout life. *Journal of Applied Physiology* 33, 805 (1972).

Ferre, C.E. amd Rand, G., The effect of increased intensity of light on the visual acuity of presbyopic and nonpresbyopic eyes. *Transactions of the Illumination Engineering Society* 29, 296 (1937).

Finch, C.E., *Longevity, Senescence, and the Genome*. University of Chicago Press, Chicago (1991).

Hughes, G., Changes in taste sensitivity with advancing age. *Gerontological Clinic*. 11, 224 (1969).

Howard, B., Growing younger. Can growth hormone make the clock run backwards? *Longevity* 4, 38 (1992).

Kay, M.M.B., An overview of immune aging. *Mechanisms of Ageing and Development* 9, 39 (1979).

Leopold, A.C., The biological significance of death in plants, in *The Biology of Aging* (J. Behnke, C. Finch, and G. Moment, editors). Plenum, New York (1978).

Maynard-Smith, J., Review lectures on senescence. I. The causes of ageing. *Proceedings of the Royal Society of London Series B*. 157, 115 (1962).

Medawar, P.B., *An Unsolved Problem in Biology*. H.K. Lewis, London (1952).

Rowe, J.W., Andres, R., Tobin, J.D., Norris, A.H., and Shock, N.W., The effect of age on creatinine clearance in man;

a cross sectional and longitudinal study. *Journal of Gerontology* 31, 155 (1976).

Rudman, D., Feller, A.G., Nagraj, H.S., and coworkers, Effects of human growth hormone in men over 60 years old. *New England Journal of Medicine* 323, 1 (1990).

Rudman, D., Feller, A.G., Cohn, L., and coworkers, Effects of human growth hormone on body composition in elderly men. *Hormone Research* 36 (Suppl 1), 73 (1991).

Shock, N.W., Physiological and chronological age, in *Aging — Its Chemistry*. (Dietz, A.A., editor). American Association for Clinical Chemistry, Washington, (1980).

Shock, N.W. and Norris, A.H., Neuromuscular coordination as a factor in age changes in exercise, in *Physical Activity and Aging*, Vol. 4 (Jokl, E. and Brunner, D., editors) Karger, Basel (1970).

Strehler, B.L., *Time, Cells, and Aging* 2nd Edition. Academic Press, New York (1977).

Walford, R., *Maximum Life Span* Norton, New York (1983).

Weiss, A.D., Auditory perception in relation to age, in *Human Aging* (Birren, J., editor) U.S. Government Printing Office, Washington (1963).

Weiss, J.S., Ellis, C.N., Headington, J.T., and coworkers, Topical trentoin improves photoaged skin. *Journal of the American Medical Association* 259, 527 (1988).

Chapter 8 — The Causes Of Aging

Armstrong, D., Rinehart, R., Dixon, L., and Reigh, D., Changes of peroxidase with age in *Drosophila. Age* 1, 8 (1978).

Bailey, P.J. and Webster, G.C., Lowered rates of protein synthesis by mitochondria isolated from organisms of increasing age. *Mechanisms of Ageing and Development* 24, 233 (1984).

Biscardi, H.M. and Webster, G.C., Accumulation of fluorescent age pigments in different genetic strains of *Drosophila melanogaster. Experimental Gerontology* 12, 201 (1977).

Blazejowski, C.A. and Webster, G.C., Decreased rates of protein synthesis by cell-free preparations from different organs of aging mice. *Mechanisms of Ageing and Development* 21, 345 (1983).

Celis, J.E., Rasmussen, H.H., Leffers, H., and coworkers, Human cellular protein patterns and their link to genome DNA sequence data: usefulness of two-dimensional gel electrophoresis and microsequencing. *FASEB Journal* 5, 2200 (1991).

Coniglio, J.J., Liu, D.S.H., and Richardson, A., A comparison of protein synthesis by liver parenchymal cells isolated from Fischer F344 rats of various ages. *Mechanisms of Ageing and Development* 11, 77 (1979).

Ekstrom, R., Liu, D.S.H., and Richardson, A., Changes in brain protein synthesis during the life span of male Fischer rats. *Gerontology* 26, 121 (1980).

Hardwick, J., Hsieh, W.H., Liu, D.S.H., and Richardson, A., Cell-free protein synthesis by kidney from the aging female Fischer 344 rat. *Biochimica et Biophysica Acta* 652, 204 (1981).

Herbener, G.H., A morphometric study of age-dependent changes in mitochondrial populations of mouse liver and heart. *Journal of Gerontology* 31, 8 (1976).

Lavie, L., Reznick, A.Z., and Gershon, D., Decreased protein and puromycinyl-peptide degradation in livers of senescent mice. *Biochemical Journal* 202, 47 (1982).

Mainwaring, W.I.P., The effect of age on protein synthesis in mouse liver. *Biochemical Journal* 113, 869 (1969).

Massie, H.R., Colacicco, J.R., and Williams, T.R., Loss of mitochondrial DNA with aging in the Swedish C strain of *Drosophila melanogaster. Age* 4, 42 (1981).

Miquel, J. and Johnson, Jr., J.E., Senescent changes in the ribosomes of animal cells in vivo and in vitro. *Mechanisms of Ageing and Development* 9, 247 (1979).

Nette, E.G., Xi, Y., Sun, Y., Andrews, A.D., and King, D.W., A correlation between aging and DNA repair in human epidermal cells. *Mechanisms of Ageing and Development* 24, 283 (1984).

O'Farrell, P.H., High resolution two-dimensional electrophoresis of proteins. *Journal of Biological Chemistry* 250, 4007 (1975).

Ono, T., Okada, S., and Sugahara, T., Comparative studies of DNA size in various tissues of mice during the aging process. *Experimental Gerontology* 11, 127 (1976).

Peterson, J.L. and McConkey, E.H., Non-histone chromosomal proteins from HeLa cells. A survey by high-resolution, two-dimensional electrophoresis. *Journal of Biological Chemistry* 251, 548 (1976).

Plesko, M. and Richardson, A., Age-related changes in unscheduled DNA synthesis by rat hepatocytes. *Biochemical and Biophysical Research Communications* 118, 730 (1984).

Price, G.B., Modak, S.P., and Makinodan, T., Age-associated changes in the DNA of mouse tissue. *Science* 171, 917 (1971).

Rao, G., Xia, E., and Richardson, A., Effect of age on the expression of antioxidant enzymes in male Fischer F344 rats. *Mechanisms of Ageing and Development* 53, 49 (1990).

Richardson, A., The relationship between aging and protein synthesis. *Handbook of Biochemistry in Aging.* (Florini, J.R., editor) CRC Press, Boca Raton, (1981).

Sonntag, W.E., Hylka, V.W., and Meites, J., Growth hormone restores protein synthesis in skeletal muscle of old male rats. *Journal of Gerontology* 40, 689 (1985).

Tappel, A.L., Fletcher, B., and Deamer, D., Effect of antioxidants and nutrients on lipid peroxidation fluorescent products and aging parameters in the mouse. *Journal of Gerontology* 28, 415 (1973).

Tauchi, M. and Sato, T., Age changes in size and number of mitochondria in human hepatic cells. *Journal of Gerontology* 23, 454 (1968).

Treff, W.M., Das Involutionsmuster des Nucleus dentatus cerebelli. In *Altern* (Platt, D., editor). Schattauer, Stuttgart (1974).

Vann, A.C. and Webster, G.C., Age-related changes in mitochondrial function in *Drosophila melanogaster. Experimental Gerontology* 12, 1 (1977).

Webster, G.C. and Webster, S.L., Decreased protein synthesis by microsomes from aging *Drosophila melanogaster. Experimental Gerontology* 14, 343 (1979).

Wilson. P.D., Enzyme levels in animals of various ages. *Handbook of Biochemistry in Aging.* (Florini, J.R., editor) CRC Press, Boca Raton, (1981).

Yu, C.E., Oshima, J., Fu, Y.H., and coworkers, Positional cloning of the Werner's syndrome gene. *Science* 272, 258 (1996).

Chapter 9 — The Search For Shangri-La

Barrett-Connor, E., Khaw, K.-T., and Yen, S.S.C., A prospective study of dehydroepiandrosterone sulfate, mortality, and cardiovascular disease. *New England Journal of Medicine* 315, 1519 (1986).

Barrows, C.H. and Kokkonen, G., The effect of dietary cellulose on life span and biochemical variables of male mice. *Age* 11, 7 (1988).

Beuchene, R.E., Bales, C.W., Bragg, C.S., Hawkins, S.T., Mason, R.L., Effect of age initiation of feed restriction on growth, body composition, and longevity of rats. *Journal of Gerontology* 41, 13 (1986).

Birchenall-Sparks, M.C., Roberts, M.S., Staecker, J., Hardwick, J.P., and Richardson, A., Effect of dietary restriction on liver protein synthesis. *Journal of Nutrition* 115, 110 (1985).

Birkmayer, W., Knoll, J., Riederer, P., and coworkers, Increased life expectancy resulting from addition of L-deprenyl to Madopar treatment in Parkinson's disease: a longterm study. *Journal of Neural Transmission* 64, 113 (1985).

Blackett, A.D. and Hall, D.A., The effects of vitamin E on mouse fitness and survival. *Gerontology* 27, 133 (1981).

Bulbrook, R.D., Hayward, J.L., and Spicer, C.C., Relation between urinary androgen and corticoid excretion and subsequent breast cancer. *Lancet* 2, 395 (1971).

Cheney, K.E., Liu, R.K., Smith, G.S., and coworkers, The effect of dietary restriction of varying duration on survival, tumor patterns, immune function, and body temperature in B10C3F1 mice. *Journal of Gerontology* 38, 420 (1983).

Chopra, D., *Ageless Body, Timeless Mind.* Harmony Books, New York (1993).

Clapp, N.K., Satterfield, L.C., and Bowles, N.D., Effects of the antioxidant butylated hydroxytoluene (BHT) on mortality in BALB/c mice. *Journal of Gerontology* 34, 497 (1979).

Cohn, R.R., Effect of antioxidants on life-span of C57Bl mice. *Journal of Gerontology* 26, 378 (1971).

Comfort, A., Youhotsky-Gore, I., and Pathmanathan, K., Effect of ethoxyquin on the longevity of C3H mice. *Nature* 229, 254 (1971).

Economos, A.C., Ballard, R.C., Miquel, J., and coworkers, Accelerated aging of fasted *Drosophila*. Preservation of physiological function and cellular fine structure by thiazolidine carboxylic acid. *Experimental Gerontology* 17, 105 (1982).

Freisleben, H.J., Lehr, F., and Fuchs, J., Lifespan of immunosuppressed NMRI-mice is increased by deprenyl. *Journal of Neural Transmission, Suppl.* 41, 231 (1994).

Harman, D., Prolongation of the normal life span by radiation protection chemicals. *Journal of Gerontology* 12, 257 (1957).

Harman, D., Prolongation of the normal lifespan and inhibition of spontaneous cancer by antioxidants. *Journal of Gerontology* 16, 247 (1961).

Harman, D., Free radical theory of aging: effect of free radical reaction inhibitors on the mortality rate of male LAF mice. *Journal of Gerontology* 23, 476 (1968).

Harman, D., Free radical theory of aging: effect of free radical inhibitors on the life span of male LAF mice — second experiment. *Gerontologist* 8, 13 (1968).

Harrison, D.E., Archer, J.R., and Astle, C.M., Effects of food restriction on aging: separation of food intake and adiposity. *Proceedings of the National Academy of Sciences USA* 81, 1835 (1984).

Hochschild, R., Effect of membrane stabilizing drugs on mortality in *Drosophila melanogaster*. *Experimental Gerontology* 6, 133 (1971).

Hochschild, R., Effect of dimethylaminoethyl parachlorophenoxyacetate on the life span of male Swiss Webster mice. *Experimental Gerontology* 8, 177 (1973).

Hochschild, R., The H-Scan — an instrument for automatic measurement of physiological markers of aging. *Intervention in the Aging Process* (Regelson, W. and Sinex, F.M., editors) Alan R. Liss, New York (1983).

Kitani, K., Kanai, S., Sato, Y., Ohta, M., and others, Chronic treatment of (-) deprenyl prolongs the life span of male Fischer 344 rats. *Life Science* 52, 281 (1993).

Knoll, J., The striatal dopamine dependency of life span in male rats. Longevity study with (-)deprenyl. *Mechanisms of Ageing and Development* 46, 237 (1988).

Knoll, J., Dallo, J., and Yen, T.T., Striatal dopamine, sexual activity, and lifespan. Longevity of rats treated with (-)deprenyl. *Life Sciences* 45, 525 (1989).

McCay, C.M., Crowell, M.F., and Maynard, L.A., The effect of retarded growth upon the length of life span and upon ultimate body size. *Journal of Nutrition* 10, 63 (1935).

Migeon, C.J., Keller, A.R., Lawrence, B., and Shepard, T.H., Dehydroepiandrosterone and androsterone levels in human plasma. Effect of age and sex; day-to-day and diurnal variations. *Journal of Clinical Endocrinology and Metabolism* 17, 1051 (1957).

Milgram, N.W., Racine, R.J., Nellis, P., Mendonca, A, and Ivy, G.O., Maintenance on L-deprenyl prolongs life in aged male rats. *Life Sciences* 47, 415 (1990).

Miquel, J. and Economos, A.C., Favorable effects of the antioxidants sodium and magnesium thiazolidine carboxylate on the vitality and life span of *Drosophila* and mice. *Experimental Gerontology* 14, 279 (1979).

Mollen, A. and Sachs, J., *Doctor Mollen's Anti-Aging Diet.* Penguin, New York (1993).

Nandy, K. and Bourne, G.H., Effect of centrophenoxine on the lipofuscin pigments in the neurones of senile guinea pigs. *Nature* 210, 313 (1966).

Pearson, D. and Shaw, S., *Life Extension*. Warner, New York (1982).

Richardson, A., The effect of age and nutrition on protein synthesis by cells and tissues from mammals. In *Handbook of Nutrition in the Aged*. (Watson, R.R., editor) CRC Press, Boca Raton (1985).

Sawada, M. and Enesco, H.E., Vitamin E extends lifespan in the short-lived rotifer *Asplanchna brightwelli*. *Experimental Gerontology* 19, 179 (1984).

Schneider, E.H. and Reed, J.D., Life extension. *New England Journal of Medicine* 312, 1159 (1985).

Schwartz, A.G., Pashko, L.L., and Tannen, R.H., Dehydroepiandrosterone: an anti-cancer and possible anti-aging substance. *Intervention in the Aging Process* Regelson, W. and Sinex, F.M., editors) Alan R. Liss, Inc., New York (1983).

Shlian, D.M. and Goldstone, J., Toxicity of butylated hydroxytoluene. *New England Journal of Medicine* 314, 648 (1986)

Walford, R.L., *Maximum Life Span* Norton New York (1983).

Yu, B.P., Masoro, E.J., Murata, I., Bertrand, H.A., and Lynd, F.T., Life span study of SPF Fischer 344 male rats fed ad libitum or restricted diets: Longevity, growth, lean body mass, and disease. *Journal of Gerontology* 37, 130 (1982).

Zuckerman, B.M. and Geist, M.A., Effects of vitamin E on the nematode *Caenorhabditis elegans*. *Age* 6, 1 (1983).

Chapter 10 — The Highway To Immortality

Arking, R. and Clare, M., Genetics of aging: effective selection for increased longevity in *Drosophila*. *Insect Aging*. (Collatz, K.G. and Sohal, R.S., editors) Springer-Verlag, Berlin (1986).

Bell, A.G., *The Duration of Life and Conditions Associated with Longevity. A Study of the Hyde Genealogy*. Private printing. Washington, D.C., (1918).

Blazejowski, C.A. and Webster, G.C., Effect of age on peptide chain initiation and elongation in preparations from brain, liver, kidney, and skeletal muscle of the C57Bl/6J mouse. *Mechanisms of Ageing and Development* 25, 323 (1984).

Cavallius, J., Rattan, S.I.S., and Clark, B.F.C., Changes in activity and amount of of active elongation factor 1a in ageing and immortal human fibroblast cultures. *Experimental Gerontology* 21, 149 (1986).

Cristofalo, V.J., Animal cell cultures as a model system for the study of aging. *Advances in Gerontological Research* 4, 45 (1972).

Derventzi, A., Rattan, S.I., and Clark, B.F., Phorbol ester PMA stimulates protein synthesis and increases the levels of active elongation factors EF-1 alpha and EF-2 in ageing human fibroblasts. *Mechanisms of Ageing and Development* 69, 193 (1993).

Dimri, G.P. and Campisi, J., Transcriptional control of cellular replicative senescence. *Molecular Biology of the Cell* 5, 386a (1994).

D'mello, N.P., Childress, A.M., Franklin, D.S., Kale, S.P., and others, Cloning and characterization of LAG1, a longevity-assurance gene in yeast. *Journal of Biological Chemistry*, 269, 15451 (1994).

Ebert, R.H., Cherkasova, V.A., Dennis, R.A., Wu, J.H., and others, Longevity-determining genes in *Caenorhabditis elegans*: chromosomal mapping of multiple noninteractive loci. *Genetics* 135, 1003 (1993).

Engelhardt, D.L., Lee, G.T.Y., and Moley, J.F., Patterns of peptide synthesis in senescent and presenescent human fibroblasts. *Journal of Cellular Physiology* 98, 193 (1979).

Friedmann, H., Progress toward human gene therapy. *Science* 244, 1275 (1989).

Gabius, H.J., Goldbach, S, Graupner, G., Rehm, S. and Cramer, F., Organ pattern of age-related changes in the aminoacyl-tRNA synthetase activities of the mouse. *Mechanisms of Ageing and Development* 20, 305 (1982).

Gabius, H.J., Engelhardt, R., Deerberg, F., and Cramer, F., Age-related changes in different steps of protein synthesis of liver and kidney of rats. *FEBS Letters* 160, 115 (1983).

Goldstein, S., Replicative senescence: the human fibroblast comes of age. *Science* 249, 1129 (1990).

Gonzalez, B.M., Experimental studies on the duration of life. VIII. The influence upon duration of life of certain mutant genes of *Drosophila melanogaster. American Naturalist* 57, 289 (1923).

Harley, C.B., Futcher, A.B., and Greider, C.W., Telomeres shorten during ageing of human fibroblasts. *Nature* 345, 458 (1990).

Hayflick, L., The limited in vitro lifetime of human diploid cell strains. *Experimental Cell Research* 37, 614 (1965).

Hayflick, L. and Moorhead, P.S., The serial cultivation of human diploid cell strains. *Experimental Cell Research* 25, 585 (1961).

Heydari, A.R, Wu, B., Takahashi, R., Strong, R., and Richardson, A., Expression of heat shock protein 70 is altered by age and diet at the level of transcription. *Molecular and Cellular Biology* 13, 2909 (1993).

Hung, L. and Richardson, A., The effect of aging on the genetic expression of renin by mouse kidney. *Aging* (Milano) 5, 193 (1993).

Jazwinski, S.M., The genetics of aging in the yeast *Saccharomyces cerevisiae. Genetica* 91, 35 (1993).

Johnson, T.E., Increased life-span of age-1 mutants of *Caenorhabditis elegans* and lower Gompertz rate of aging. *Science* 249, 908 (1990).

Johnson, T.E., Tedesco, P.M., and Lithgow, G.J., Comparing mutants, selective breeding, and transgenics in the dissection of aging processes of *Caenorhabditis elegans*. *Genetica* 91, 65 (1993).

Kenyon, C., Chang, J., Gensch, E., Rudner, A., and Tabtiang, R., A *C. elegans* mutant that lives twice as long as wild type. *Nature* 366, 461 (1993).

Kim, N.W., Piatyszek, M.A., Prowse, K.R., and coworkers, Specific association of human telomerase activity with immortal cells and cancer. *Science* 266, 2011 (1994).

Larsen, P.L., Aging and resistance to oxidative damage in *Caenorhabditis elegans*. *Proceedings of the National Academy of Sciences, U.S.* 90, 8905 (1993).

Larsen, P.L., Albert, P.S., and Riddle, D.L., Genes that regulate both development and longevity in *Caenorhabditis elegans*. *Genetics* 139, 1567 (1995).

Laskowski, B. and Hekimi, S., Determination of life-span in Caenorhabditis elegans by four clock genes. Science 272, 1010 (1996).

Maier, J.A.M., Voulalas, P., Roeder, D., and Maciag, T., Extension of the life-span of human endothelial cells by an interleukin-1a antisense oligomer. *Science* 249, 1570 (1990).

Moldave, K., Harris, J., Sabo, W., and Sadnik, I., Protein synthesis and aging: studies with cell-free systems. *Federation Proceedings* 38, 1979 (1979).

Nagy, I.Z. and Semsei, I., Centrophenoxine increases the rates of total and mRNA synthesis in the brain cortex of old rats. *Experimental Gerontology* 19, 171 (1984).

Orr, W.C. and Sohal, R.S., Extension of life-span by overexpression of superoxide dismutase and catalase in *Drosophila melanogaster. Science* 263, 1128 (1994).

Pearl, R. and Miner, J.R., Experimental studies on the duration of life. XIV. The comparative mortality of certain lower organisms. *Quarterly Review of Biology* 10, 60 (1935).

Rao, G., Xia, E., and Richardson, A., Effect of age on the expression of antioxidant enzymes in male Fischer F344 rats. *Mechanisms of Ageing and Development* 53, 49 (1990).

Richardson, A., Rutherford, M.S., Birchenall-Sparks, M.C., and coworkers, Levels of specific messenger RNA species as a function of age. *Molecular Biology of Aging* (Sohal, R., Birnbaum, L., and Cutler, R., editors) Raven Press, New York (1985).

Rockstein, M., The genetic basis for longevity. *Theoretical Aspects of Aging.* (Rockstein, M., Sussman, M.L., and Chesky, J., editors) Academic Press, New York (1974).

Rose, M.R., Laboratory evolution of postponed senescence in *Drosophila melanogaster. Evolution* 38, 1004 (1984).

Seshadri, T. and Campesi, J., Repression of c-fos transcription and an altered genetic program in senescent human fibroblasts. *Science* 247, 205 (1990).

Seshadri, T, Uzman, J.A., Oshima, J. and Campisi, J., Identification of a transcript that is down-regulated in senescent human fibroblasts. *Journal of Biological Chemistry* 268, 18474 (1993).

Shepherd, J.C.W., Walldorf, U., Hug, P., and Gehring, W., Fruit flies with additional expression of elongation factor EF-1a live longer. *Proceedings of the National Academy of Sciences of the U.S.* 86, 7520 (1989).

Silar, P. and Picard, M., Increased longevity of EF-1 alpha high-fidelity mutants in Podospora anserina. *Journal of Molecular Biology* 235, 231 (1994).

Smith, J.R. and Pereira-Smith, O.M., Further studies on the genetic and biochemical basis of cellular senescence. *Experimental Gerontology* 24, 377 (1989).

Webster, G.C., Protein synthesis in aging organisms. *Molecular Biology of Aging* (Sohal, R., Birnbaum, L., and Cutler, R., editors) Raven Press, New York (1985).

Webster, G.C., Protein synthesis. *Drosophila as a Model Organism for Ageing Studies.* (Lints, F. and Soliman, M., Editors) Blackie Publishers, Glasgow (1987).

Webster, G.C. and Webster, S.L., Aminoacylation of tRNA by cell-free preparations from aging *Drosophila melanogaster. Experimental Gerontology* 16, 487 (1981).

Webster, G.C. and Webster, S.L., Effects of age on the post initiation stages of protein synthesis. *Mechanisms of Ageing and Development* 18, 369 (1982).

Webster, G.C. and Webster, S.L., Specific disappearance of translatable messenger RNA for elongation factor one in aging *Drosophila melanogaster. Mechanisms of Ageing and Development* 24, 335 (1984).

Webster, G.C., Webster, S.L., and Landis, W.A., The effect of age on the initiation of protein synthesis in *Drosophila melanogaster. Mechanisms of Ageing and Development* 16, 71 (1981).

Wimonwatwatee, T., Heydari, A.R., Wu, W.T. and Richardson, A., Effect of age on the expression of phosphoenolpyruvate carboxykinase in rat liver. *American Journal of Physiology* 267, G201 (1994).

Wu, W.T., Pahlavani, M., Cheung, H.T., and Richardson, A., The effect of aging on the expression of interleukin-2 messenger ribonucleic acid. *Cellular Immunology* 100, 224 (1986).

Chapter 11 — Changing The Course Of History

Butler, R.N., *Why Survive? Being Old in America.* Harper, New York (1975).

Callahan, D., *Setting Limits: Medical Costs in an Aging Society.* Simon and Schuster, New York (1987).

Daniels, N., *Am I My Parents' Keeper? An Essay on Justice Between the Young and the Old.* Oxford, New York (1988).

Fries, J.F., Koop, C.E., Beadle, C.F., and the Health Project Consortium, Reducing health care costs by reducing the need and demand for medical services. *New England Journal of Medicine* 329, 321 (1993).

Gates, B., *The Road Ahead.* Viking, New York (1995).

Gori, G.B., Richter, B.J., and Yu, W.K., Economics and extended longevity: a case study. *Preventive Medicine* 13, 396 (1984).

Iglehart, J.K., Medical care of the poor — a growing problem. *New England Journal of Medicine* 313, 59 (1985).

Koltikoff, L.J., Some economic implications of life span extension. *Aging: Biology and Behavior* (J. March, J.L. McGaugh and S.B. Keisler, editors) Academic Press, New York (1982).

Levinsky, N.G., Age as a criterion for rationing health care. *New England Journal of Medicine* 322, 1813 (1990).

Markley, O.and McCuan, W., *21st Century Earth.* Greenhaven Press, San Diego (1996).

Scott, H.D. and Shapiro, H.B., Universal insurance for American health care. A proposal of the American College of Physicians. *Annals of Internal Medicine* 117, 511 (1992).

Vagelos, P.R., Are prescription drug prices high? *Science* 252, 1080 (1991).

Walford, R.L., *Maximum Life Span*. Norton, New York (1983).

Chapter 12 — The Future

Clark, A.C., *Profiles of the Future*. Harper and Row, New York (1963).

Fisher, J.A., *Rx 2000: Breakthroughs in Health, Medicine, and Longevity*. Simon and Schuster, New York (1992).

Friedmann, H., Progress toward human gene therapy. *Science* 244, 1275 (1989).

Naisbitt, J., *Megatrends*. Warner, New York (1982).

Toffler, A., *The Third Wave*. Morrow, New York (1980).

Watson, J.D., The human genome project: past, present, and future. *Science* 248, 44 (1990).

Index

About the Author

George Webster is a research scientist, lecturer, and analyst of future trends. A recognized authority on aging, he has published nearly a hundred reports in scientific journals on his discoveries about the causes of aging and on related topics in molecular biology.

Previously, he served as a Senior Research Fellow at Cal Tech, a Professor of Biochemistry at Ohio State, a Visiting Professor at the University of Wisconsin, an Established Investigator of the American Heart Association, and Head of Biological Sciences at Florida Tech. Webster was also chief of the Medical Department's Environmental Health Labratory at Cape Canaveral and served in the US Air Force as a combat flyer.

George Webster is a Fellow of the American Association for the Advancement of Science, and a member of the American Society for Biochemistry and Molecular Biology, American Society for Cell Biology, and the Society of the Sigma Xi. He lives in central Florida.

Addicus Books

Visit the Addicus Books Web Site
http://members.aol.com/addicusbks

Hello, Methuselah! Living to 100 and Beyond	*$14.95*
George Webster ISBN 1-886039-259	
The Family Compatibility Test	*$9.95*
Susan Adams ISBN 1-886039-27-5	
First Impressions — Tips to Enhance Your Image	*$14.95*
Joni Craighead ISBN 1-886039-26-7	
Straight Talk About Breast Cancer	*$9.95*
Susan Braddock, MD ISBN 1-886039-21-6	
Prescription Drug Abuse — The Hidden Epidemic	*$14.95*
Rod Colvin ISBN 1-886030-22-4	
The Healing Touch — Keeping the Doctor/ Patient Relationship Alive Under Managed Care	*$9.95*
David Cram, MD ISBN 1-886039-31-3 (Fall 1997)	
The ABCs of Gold Investing	*$14.95*
Michael J. Kosares ISBN 1-886039-29-1	
The Flat Tax: Why It Won't Work for America	*$12.95*
Scott E. Hicko ISBN 1-886039-28-3	

Please send:

_____ copies of_____

(*Title of book*)

at $ _____each   TOTAL   _____

Nebr. residents add 5% sales tax   _____

Shipping/Handling
  $3.00 for first book.
  $1.00 for each additional book.   _____

TOTAL ENCLOSED   _____

Name_____

Address_____

City _____ State____ Zip _____

☐ Visa ☐ Master Card ☐ Am. Express

Credit card number _____

Expiration date _____

Order by credit card, personal check or money order.
Send to:

Addicus Books
Mail Order Dept.
P.O. Box 45327
Omaha, NE 68145
Or, order **TOLL FREE: 800-352-2873**